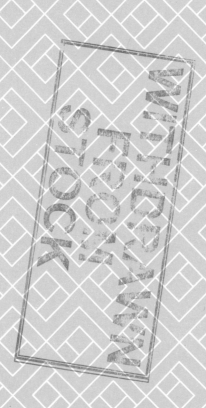

Making social work news

Social work has recently received some dreadful news coverage, but the most extravagant headlines and accusations centre on local authority social work with children. Moreover, they are almost exclusively from the national press.

In *Making Social Work News*, Meryl Aldridge widens the debate on social work and its representation by the news media. The book falls into three parts, the first providing students and practitioners with a basic understanding of the day-to-day working and commercial logic of the UK press. The second part examines the press coverage of social work itself, exploring its considerable variation, comparing different news treatments between broadsheets and tabloids, and between national and local papers. The final part considers whether social work has particular difficulties in defining its goals and lobbying on its own behalf. It concludes with some reflections on the importance of doing so now that marketing has become part of the policy process.

Making Social Work News will be invaluable to all students and lecturers in social work, sociology and social policy as well as media and cultural studies. It will also be essential reading for all social work professionals, particularly those involved in training.

Meryl Aldridge is Senior Lecturer in Social Studies at the University of Nottingham.

Making social work news

Meryl Aldridge

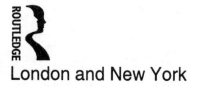

London and New York

First published in 1994
by Routledge
11 New Fetter Lane, London EC4P 4EE

Simultaneously published in the USA and Canada
by Routledge
29 West 35th Street, New York, NY 10001

Typeset in Times by
NWL Editorial Services, Langport, Somerset

Printed and bound in Great Britain by
Biddles Ltd, Guildford and King's Lynn

British Library Cataloguing in Publication Data
A catalogue record for this book is available from the British
Library

Library of Congress Cataloging in Publication Data
A catalog record for this book has been requested

ISBN 0–415–07441–X

For Alan Aldridge

Contents

Acknowledgements

This study was supported by a grant from the University of Nottingham Research Fund, supplemented by the School of Social Studies.

An earlier version of Chapter 5 appeared as an article in the *British Journal of Social Work*. The permission of the editorial board and of Oxford University Press is gratefully acknowledged.

Newspaper material for the study was collected from the British Library Newspaper Library at Colindale (truly a jewel in our heritage) and the Centre for Mass Communications Research at the University of Leicester. I would like to thank the staff at both for their willing assistance and efficiency.

Despite the pressures on them, staff involved in media relations at ACOP, NAPO, NACRO, the NSPCC, ChildLine, and two probation services in the Midlands and the south-west of England gave up time to talk to me, answer follow-up enquiries and, in some cases, collect and send me material through the post. I hope that they recognize at least some of their objectives and activities in these pages and I thank them for their contribution to my research.

Before becoming Chief Probation Officer of Warwickshire John Pendleton was, for several years, Senior Lecturer in charge of the social work course at the University of Nottingham. He died in 1989. Together with many others, I remember him as representing all that is best in professional social work.

I would like to thank all my colleagues in the School of Social Studies for co-operating in the programme of study-leave which made it possible for a major writing project to be enjoyable as well as demanding. Many of them also allowed their bookshelves and files to be raided, and gave help when faced with apparently haphazard requests for factual information or the testing out of less-than-half-formed ideas.

The following provided a wide variety of essentials – encouragement, resources, intellectual stimulation, advice, companionship, hospitality and other practical assistance: Alan Aldridge; Helen Carpenter; Peter Carpenter; Dido; Robert Dingwall; Heather Gibson; Nicki James; Pete Lowenstein; Mark Lymbery; Chris Smith; Olive Stevenson. They, and all other friends and colleagues, are partially responsible for what follows, but should not be included in the search for blame.

Nottingham, January 1994

Abbreviations and glossary

ACOP	Association of Chief Officers of Probation
ADSS	Association of Directors of Social Services
BASW	British Association of Social Workers
CCETSW	Central Council for Education and Training in Social Work
CPO	Chief Probation Officer
DoH	Department of Health
DSS	Department of Social Security
editorial	statement of the newspaper's opinion (see leader) *or* all content other than paid-for advertising, particularly in magazines
FT	the *Financial Times*
lead	the main article on a page, thus second lead, third lead, etc.
leader	editorial comment representing opinion of newspaper; may be more than one, so first leader, second leader, etc.
NACRO	National Association for the Care and Resettlement of Offenders
NALGO	National Association of Local Government Officers (now part of Unison)
NAPO	National Association of Probation Officers
news management	attempts by the subject to control their news coverage
NAYPIC	National Association of Young People in Care
NISW	National Institute of Social Work
NSPCC	National Society for the Prevention of Cruelty to Children
NUM	National Union of Mineworkers
NUPE	National Union of Public Employees (now part of Unison)
placed news	news originated by its subject
PR	public relations, also called media relations or external relations

QC	Queen's Counsel
SSI	Social Services Inspectorate (of DoH)
standfirst	highlighted introductory paragraph, outlining contents of article
starburst	irregular star-shaped background for brief exclamatory headings; favoured by mass tabloids
strapline	subsidiary headline above main headline, introducing, explaining or gathering together article(s) below
UDM	Union of Democratic Mineworkers
white-on-black (WOB)	dramatic style of presenting headline, particularly popular with mass tabloids

Introduction

THE CONTEXT

Social work has been the subject of some memorably dreadful press coverage: 'We asked for a babysitter and they sent us a monster' (*Daily Express* two-page splash headline, 18 December 1984, on the trial of Colin Evans); 'BLUNDERS THAT LED TO BABY'S MURDER' (*Sun* p. 1, 26 July 1985, on the Tyra Henry inquiry report); 'Such awesome powers would be the envy of many a totalitarian state' (*Daily Mail* leader, 15 September 1990, on the Rochdale wardship proceedings); 'Social workers lashed as "Satan kids" are set free' (*Daily Mirror* p. 1 headline, 8 March 1991, on the Rochdale judgement).

Since the furore over the Maria Colwell trial in 1973 and the subsequent public inquiry, British social workers have been convinced that any policy dispute or practice error will produce news reports ranging from poorly informed to systematically excoriating. No sooner had the anxieties of the 1970s subsided than a series of trials in the mid-1980s reopened the issue. Once more named individuals were portrayed as having allowed a preventable death. Then, in 1987, the Cleveland child sex abuse events fired another major controversy, repeated in similar forms in Rochdale and the Orkneys. Social workers were accused of being suggestible and gullible, of assembling unrelated symptoms or childish imaginings into fantastic edifices of abuse.

So far, so familiar; much has been published about the media images of social work. Practitioners, mostly writing in the profession's trade press, have concentrated on the experiential and the practical: the anguish of being pursued and accused; how social services can parley with the press. Friendly journalists have pointed out how unrealistic, ill-organized and incoherent social workers can be when faced with media enquiries, and proceeded to offer expert advice. Academic commentators have drawn attention to the complexity of social work's relationship with the family and the state, especially during a period of savage retrenchment in public spending. Inevitably, perhaps, most of these accounts centred on the worst of the coverage: the mass tabloids at their most raucous; the mid-market press at its most paranoid; the broadsheets handing down sententious *ex cathedra* judgements with a variety of political inflections. Much of the commentary has had a pained, breathless, 'my goodness, have you seen this?' quality.

THE DEVELOPMENT AND METHODS OF THE STUDY

In the early 1970s I joined what is now the School of Social Studies to provide sociology teaching for students on the postgraduate social work qualifying course. I was, therefore, a close observer of these cycles of agitation and relative tranquillity about social work's relations with the news media. My own interest in newsmaking, semi-dormant from student journalism days, began to intensify to the extent that it became my main teaching and research focus.

As my involvement grew, so did my concern to try and widen out the debate on the construction of social work news. Two destructive processes were feeding each other. First, social work professionals were applying little theorized understanding either of the way the news media work or of their location in the social structure. They shared the lay tendency to refer to 'the media', without distinguishing between broadcast news and the press, between the market sectors of the press (newspapers are a precision-engineered product), or between local and national media, with their very different professional and commercial imperatives. Moreover, the occupational ideology of media personnel, from junior reporter to editor-in-chief, was being accepted uncritically. News organizations' claims about autonomy and their fearless search for positivist 'truth' were taken literally; that the politics and financing of news media are inscribed in their messages was frequently overlooked.

Second, the constant reference to the same instances of partial, hysterical, and sometimes downright malevolent news coverage perpetuated a powerful unstated assumption. Social workers' very real fears were being fuelled with the notion that, anywhere, any time, any controversy over practice with every type of case or client group, by every agency, would always be given the same grotesque news treatment in every sector of the news media as in these examples. Manifestly it is not.

The study therefore has three linked objectives.

• To explore the variation that exists even in the reporting of that part of social work that has, in reality, been at the epicentre of hostile coverage: local authority work with children and families. Did all culpable deaths of children known to the local authority get the same intensity of coverage? What about the accounts of social services' involvement in cases of suspected or proven cases of non-fatal child abuse? How did the media react when the abuser was a social services employee?

- To compare the different forms of news treatment between the various national newspapers and between the national and the local press.
- To examine news media accounts of social work by agencies other than local authority social services, and also with clients of social services other than children and families.

The data collected to support the discussion were, as always, largely governed by the resources available. Archives of broadcast news exist, but access to them is difficult and/or expensive. Assembling such material afresh is very expensive. Newspapers were the obvious choice. As I was collecting the data myself I had to try to make maximum use of the research time allegedly available to the holders of teaching posts in the modern university.

Reading old newspapers is great fun, but alarmingly slow. Rather than, say, trying to conduct a complete search for a period of time, I decided to construct a sample of social work episodes for scrutiny. (Where the events were long-drawn-out, key developments were identified.) Some of these were very well known. Here, the aim was to demonstrate the diversity of coverage in scale, scope and tone. Others were instances where reporting had been very limited or non-existent. These were equally important: a key part of my methodology was to pursue the question 'what does *not* make the news?'

Reading all the newspapers was also not feasible so, for most of the case studies, I applied the following sampling frame to the range of UK national daily newspapers (not including the Sunday papers, which have a different news agenda): a Conservative-orientated broadsheet (more often the *Daily Telegraph* than *The Times*); a centre-to-left broadsheet (the *Guardian* or *The Independent* – the latter post-dated some of the earlier cases); a mid-market tabloid (more often the *Daily Mail* than the *Daily Express*, as the *Mail* is the market leader and has a consuming interest in social work; *Today*, although it has an interesting history, is relatively insignificant); the *Sun* (as Tory mass tabloid and a major social phenomenon, not the *Daily Star*, which is an also-ran in the same market sector); the *Daily Mirror* as the Labour-supporting mass tabloid.

The comparison with local newspaper accounts of social work was made through a three-month collection of the Nottingham *Evening Post*; all the *Evening Post* coverage of a major local welfare issue; the Oldham *Evening Chronicle*'s perspective on the Charlene Salt case; the *Leicester Mercury*'s reporting of the Frank Beck trial; and the local/regional newspaper clippings of a probation service in the south-west of England.

As well as the raw data from newspapers, I also collected publicity material from a number of probation service agencies and voluntary organizations, and interviewed their staff member handling media relations.

• In summary, the empirical core of the study is the treatment of a selected set of social work episodes and controversies in the news pages of a sample of UK national daily papers, plus the accounts in local newspapers of a sub-set of these and some further instances, plus interview material from a small number of media relations staff in the probation and voluntary social work sectors, plus publicity material and records from those agencies. The research is entirely about representations, not about what 'really happened'. On the contrary: I do not in any way endorse the truth of the newspaper accounts used, and have also tried to avoid taking any position on the competing accounts of the events described.

During the course of the data collection and interviews, my fascination with the issues and the research possibilities has continued. There is so much more that could be studied, for example: television and radio news, current affairs, and drama presentation of social work issues; the non-news pages of the national press where editorial, readers' letters, features and deliberately infuriating columnists are orchestrated together; the general-interest women's magazines and their information on and interpretation of social welfare issues; a longitudinal study of a social services department – or other organization – to locate and interpret why some incidents which could have been newsworthy never enter the frame; interviews with key media personnel to investigate their orientation towards and understanding of contemporary social work policy and practice. Here is a meeting of the interests of practitioners and academics, of social work and media studies, and of the development of concepts and their daily use. I hope others will want to join the debate – and that research funders will see the value of enabling them do so.

THE PLAN OF THE BOOK

Chapter 1 sketches the state of the UK press; the legal framework within which the newspapers work; current thinking about media effects on the audience; the way news is identified, gathered, processed and presented; some elements of journalists' occupational culture; how different theoretical assumptions can produce fundamentally different explanations of media functioning and messages, using the idea of the 'moral panic' as an illustration.

Chapter 2, the first of the case material section, looks in detail at the coverage of the Tyra Henry trial and inquiry report. This was selected as one of the cluster of heavily publicized cases in 1984–5. (Of these Jasmine Beckford is the best known but already the subject of useful analysis.) The next case examined is the almost contemporary, heavily reported, but very differently treated, Charlene Salt case. The final part of the chapter covers a series of trials between 1985 and 1991. All followed the death of a child where there had been some social services involvement. Many of these cases appeared to have the same ingredients for dramatic news treatment as those where the child's name has become symbolic of the profession's fear of the news media. Yet they were reported very differently – why?

Chapter 3 considers three instances of the suspected or actual non-fatal abuse of children and young people: the Rochdale satanic abuse events; the condemnation of 'pin-down' methods of discipline in Staffordshire County Council children's homes; and the trial of Frank Beck for the sexual abuse of young people in his care, and some colleagues, while working for Leicestershire Social Services. The latter two were major and unequivocal failures of social services management, so how should we interpret the fact that Rochdale was the subject of the most sustained and high-pitched media attention?

Chapter 4 probes the invisibility in the news of elderly people as social work clients. The first section discusses three instances in which social services departments were actually or possibly at fault, yet did not become nationally newsworthy. In contrast, the proposed closure of Nottinghamshire elderly persons' homes was the basis of a vigorous local press campaign. The representations of the residents, and the framing of the affair as political conflict rather than social work policy failure, make a telling contrast with the reporting of child protection in the national press.

Chapter 5 investigates the media coverage of the only instance where probation work has been the subject of widespread hostile press comment

– the trial of Colin Evans for the murder of Marie Payne. Otherwise, the
probation service has been marked by its absence from the news. Since
the late 1980s there has been political pressure on the service to seek
publicity. This process is analysed, together with the resulting strategies
and successes of ACOP, NAPO and two local probation services. A final
section reflects on the prospects for the probation service's attempts to
harness the news media.

Chapter 6 looks for social work constructed as 'good news', and finds
some favourable treatment when local authorities have been involved in
supporting the victims of disasters. Routine local press coverage too can
be reasonably positive, at least in terms of not oversimplifying issues and
of ascribing to social work professionals the status of the expert voice.
The best social work news is, though, in the coverage of the voluntary
sector – where many organizations must have good and active media
relations or face collapse. Even here, though, radicalism is not acceptable
to some sections of the press, as the comparison of NACRO, NSPCC and
ChildLine shows.

Chapter 7 opens the third section of the study. How do social workers
talk to each other about their media treatment? The assumptions of
articles written by practitioners for an audience of colleagues are
unpicked, together with the related genre of 'how to deal with the
problem'. The conclusion is that social workers tend to conceive of
journalists as much less constrained than they really are, and to be
correspondingly puzzled by misrepresentation. This sense of undeserved
attack is, it is further argued, amplified by the enduring centrality of use
of self as the main tool of social work practice. The concept of 'emotional
labour' – of which social work is a particularly intense form – is then set
out. Taking these features together with the difficulty of demonstrating
'success' explains social work's high sensitivity to media criticism.

Chapter 8 pursues the question of why social work has not be able to
develop the defensive strategies of the professional formation. It
concludes that the necessary focus, a more or less consensual cognitive
base, has never stabilized. This is the outcome of direct government
determination of what constitutes 'social work' for most practitioners
through control over the responsibilities of the dominant sector, local
authority social services. Social work as 'women's work' is then debated.
The concluding section of the chapter is a brief review of the limited data
available on public attitudes to social work.

Chapter 9, in conclusion, re-examines the extent of the supposed
problem of social work's media coverage. The very real fears of
practitioners, it suggests, have been generated by a set of events that was

dramatic, vivid and painful, not only for those caught up in them but for the profession as a whole. Those events were, however, nearly all related to local authority work with children and families – and the memorably intemperate coverage was largely limited to a predicable set of newspapers which are hostile to state welfare. Reflecting on this should assist social workers and their representatives to keep the threat in perspective. Finally, it is asserted that local authority social services will have to join other public sector organizations in the self-promotion business, and some suggestions are made as to how this might be pursued. A strategy to handle unwelcome media attention, and promotional work to try and ensure that both newsgatherers and the public hear something of successful social services work are both needed. Together they could enable departments and their staff to be more at ease with the news media.

Part I

News and newspapers

Chapter 1

How the press works

MARKETS, OWNERSHIP AND FINANCE

The press is still a vital force in the UK. Despite expanding radio and television, a deep recession, and the long list of failed ventures, newspapers retain enough social and political importance for new titles to be started. In mid-1992, for instance, there was a sudden expansion of the regional Sunday paper market. Eleven weekday morning papers have national coverage; there are regional morning papers covering Wales, Scotland, Northern Ireland and parts of England, as well as local evening and morning papers, local weekly paid-for papers and local weekly free papers. Together with Sunday papers the 1988 total was 921 (Franklin and Murphy 1991: 5).

The eleven national daily papers are often referred to as 'broadsheet' or 'tabloid'. While these are technically only sizes of paper, 'broadsheet' signifies serious, high-income readership, lower sales, but more influence. This group includes the *Daily Telegraph*, the *Guardian*, *The Times*, *The Independent*, and the *Financial Times*, and is sometimes alternatively known as the 'quality' press. But this depends where you stand and what are your canons of success: Kelvin MacKenzie, successful and abrasive former editor of the *Sun*, prefers to describe the *Guardian* as the World's Worst Newspaper (Chippindale and Horrie 1990: 113).

'Tabloid' papers fall into two groups: the *Daily Mail*, the *Daily Express* and *Today* are often referred to as 'mid-market' papers, serving people with middle incomes. Although livelier typographically than the broadsheets, they contain longer and more complex news and feature items than the *Sun*, the *Daily Mirror/Daily Record* (the Scottish sister paper) and the *Daily Star*. Sometimes called the 'popular' press, this group is often simply – but confusingly – known as 'the tabloids'. For clarity I shall refer to them as the 'mass tabloids', even though the *Daily*

Star, with an October 1993 circulation of 754,022 is not in the same league as the *Sun* (3,788,312) or the *Daily Mirror* (2,570,882 without the *Daily Record*).

All the national papers except *The Independent* are parts of larger groups, in some cases huge transnational conglomerates with diverse non-newspaper and non-publishing interests. There is also extensive cross-ownership of media covering other national newspapers, regional and local papers, local commercial radio and television. The highest profile in the field is of Rupert Murdoch, who owns the *Sun*, *Today*, *The Times*, the *News of the World* and the *Sunday Times*, as well as a controlling interest in British Sky Broadcasting satellite broadcasting. With a combined weekday sale of 4,793,701 and of 5,977,780 on Sundays – and the readership an unknown multiple of that figure – the social significance of his newspapers is evident, as is the potential influence of those who determine their editorial policy, although its actual impact is a matter of lively academic and public debate. (For further details of the structure of media ownership see, for example, Curran and Seaton 1991; Seymour-Ure 1991. All detailed analyses of media ownership are inevitably out of date by publication and should be used with care.)

Broadcasting in the UK, whether publicly or commercially funded, is required to be 'impartial', that is, not to take an overtly political editorial stance. There are no such limitations on the press. Most national dailies are broadly aligned with one of the three main parties. The *Daily Telegraph*, *The Times*, the *Daily Mail*, the *Daily Express*, the *Sun* and the *Daily Star* are clearly Conservative, although cleavages within the party, notably over Europe, are apparent both within and between these papers. The *Daily Mirror* remains right-wing-Labour supporting; the *Guardian* is anti-Tory, attempting to preserve some of its Liberal tradition but effectively supporting Labour. Having come close to closure, *Today* is now the weakest of the Murdoch papers. It appears to be trying to find a market among young adults who do not align themselves with any party but are concerned with social issues and the environment. (A cynic might wonder whether its non-Toryism has at least one eye on renewed political attacks on cross-media ownership, which came from all parties during the merging of Sky and British Satellite Broadcasting satellite television.) *The Independent* was set up explicitly to be non-aligned – and originally had an ownership structure designed to maintain this. Its stance is sometimes painfully 'balanced'. The *Financial Times*, on the other hand, is simply non-party and willing to attack all and sundry from its highly specialist and respected position. Given the small amount of general news in its pages, it can only just qualify as a national newspaper, and is not included in the papers sampled for the case study chapters. Among the issues it does not cover is crime/criminal justice, nor is there much consideration of social policy except in a wider political sense. The *FT* does, though, serve as a vivid illustration of the logic of newspaper funding.

At 287,811 (October 1993) the *FT* has about half the circulation of *Today*, and yet it is profitable and secure. With specialist staff and extensive overseas coverage its costs are high, but so too are the rates that it can charge its advertisers. The *FT* reaches relatively few people but they have high incomes and large material and influence resources. In this respect, the *FT* is more like a business or consumer magazine than a newspaper. These can survive on relatively small sales/readership, providing their 'niche' in the market gives advertisers access to a specialist audience with enough resources at its disposal.

Advertisers do not, on the other hand, expect readers of the *Sun* or the *Daily Mirror* typically to have high disposable incomes. The attraction of these papers is the sheer number of people that they reach. Somehow, then, the managements have to maintain and expand their slice of the market. Among the strategies used are holding down the cover price, enticing promotions like competitions, sensational (preferably exclusive) pictures and stories, and the creation of reader loyalty. *Sun* readers are frequently addressed collectively, attitudes are struck on their behalf, and they are invited to take part in joint activity, usually jingoistic and/or xenophobic such as supporting 'our boys' through placing the Union flag from page one in their window or being abusive to foreigners. (After UP YOURS DELORS on p. 1, readers were invited to go down to Dover and 'Bawl at Gaul' (*Sun* 1 November 1990).)

For broadsheet papers like the *FT*, the cover price is the less important part of their revenue; for tabloids it is significant, providing a further incentive to increase sales.

Overall newspaper sales are falling. The competition for market share is thus intense, and while it is most strident between the *Sun* and the *Daily Mirror*, the *Daily Mail* and the *Daily Express* are also in direct conflict, and *The Times*, *The Independent*, the *Daily Telegraph* and the *Guardian* are locked in a complex territorial struggle. *The Times* has lost its former standing as not only the UK's newspaper of record, but somehow above politics. All the broadsheets are now struggling simultaneously to be seen as the paper for opinion formers, while competing for the declining number of younger readers – a decline due not only to demographic trends but also to the apparent loss of the newspaper reading habit.

Newspapers have, in recent years, worked on the assumption that their readers rely on television for 'news', that is, actuality on very recent events, supported where possible by pictures/film or at least by frequently updated reports from correspondents. Survey evidence seems to support this position: Independent Television Commission research reported that between four and six times as many respondents chose television as the 'most complete', 'most accurate' and 'most fair' source of news as chose newspapers (*Spectrum*, Spring 1992).

The response of national newspapers, particularly the Sundays but increasingly those on weekdays too, has been to move to more 'comment' in the form of features about current issues and also more material on 'lifestyle': health, food, drink, fashion, personal finance, arts and other forms of consumption. Much of this is directed overtly to women readers and in many ways both content and style of address have become closer to those of women's magazines. Among the manifestations of this is an even greater focus on the personal/individual as an organizing principle of news stories, whether imputing praise or blame. And of course the 'lifestyle' features, whether upmarket or more popular, are centred on individual consumption. This does not mesh easily with the public expenditure implications of sophisticated public welfare services and therefore has important implications for the coverage of social work.

The local press remains a very strong presence in the UK for two interlocked reasons. First, there seems to be an undiminished demand for news from the immediate locality. This has been met to a lesser extent than predicted by local radio and hardly at all by television. Both the BBC and the commercial companies have regions too large for more than the occasional story to have a direct relevance for the viewer. The financial outlook for both sectors does not suggest that more resources will be devoted to local newsgathering in the foreseeable future, in either radio or television. Nor has cabled 'community television' developed in the UK as was expected. Thus local papers of all kinds provide the best and cheapest access for advertisers to a locally defined market, whether for products and services, jobs vacant or houses for sale. This is the logic behind the rapid growth of free newspapers, which, although now rationalized and in many cases absorbed by the owning group of the local 'paid-for', show little sign of disappearing even during hard economic times. (See Franklin and Murphy 1991 for a comprehensive account.)

The financial base of local papers directly affects their editorial line. Success depends upon being read by as large a proportion as possible of the local population, whatever their circumstances or affiliations. Too strong a political alignment could alienate potential buyers/readers. No doubt this, given difficult market conditions, was the thinking behind a 1991 Nottingham *Evening Post* telesales campaign, the gist of which was that the paper was no longer as unremittingly Tory as had been its reputation.

For the same reason, local papers must be more sensitive to the range and nuances of local opinion on local issues. Readers may have direct knowledge of the events, or loyalty to those involved from family networks, neighbourhood, work, ethnic or religious affiliation or leisure, providing them with the most powerful of tools to criticize media coverage. (See the discussions of media effects below and in Chapter 8.) Napoli and Napoli (1990) contrast the oversimplification of the Salman Rushdie affair in most of the UK national press with the efforts made by the *Bradford Telegraph and Argus* to reflect the range of opinions in the Muslim community. This caution about popular sentiment is also apparent in the furore over the closure of Nottinghamshire Social Services Department elderly persons' homes discussed in Chapter 4, where 'balanced' reporting of the county's financial dilemmas was gradually displaced by a noisy populist campaign.

THE PRESS AND THE LAW

Compared with those in other countries and with the broadcast media, in the UK newspapers are relatively unrestrained. Conversely, they do not have any constitutional rights to mobilize in defence of such investigative work as they undertake. This is an important difference between the press in the UK and the US; media research needs to be read in this context.

Among the principal areas of restriction on the UK press are state security, obscenity and libel. Legislation on privacy is under active consideration during 1993. The industry-run Press Complaints Commission, set up after the report of the Calcutt Committee (Cm 1102 1990), was savaged as being insufficiently independent by Sir David Calcutt in his review (Cm 2135 1993). He recommended a range of legal remedies and a statutory tribunal. A subsequent parliamentary select committee produced the compromise solution of a non-statutory Ombudsman with powers to impose financial penalties. Press reactions to this, as to the second Calcutt report, ranged from the broadsheets uttering magisterial dismissals, to mass tabloid abuse of politicians for seeking to protect their own. From the point of view of social work news, the important limitations on reporting relate to contempt of court and the involvement of children in the judicial process, whether as defendant or subject of civil proceedings.

Contempt of court is a broad concept: it includes 'publication of material which might prejudice a fair trial', 'anything which interferes with the course of justice generally', breaches of undertakings given to the court, and breaches of injunctions (Welsh and Greenwood 1992: 99). Effectively it restricts the coverage of cases in progress to a description of the proceedings, but does not rule out selectivity in which parts of them to report.

Nothing which could identify the young person(s) concerned can be reported from the proceedings of youth courts (until October 1992 juvenile courts). Powers to restrict the publication of identifying details of young persons appearing in crown courts are also usually invoked. These powers cannot, though, be used to suppress the names of defendants in child battery or sexual abuse criminal cases. In 1991 a judgement left it to the editorial decision of newspapers whether information published about defendants would enable readers to name the child concerned (Welsh and Greenwood 1992: 36). The ADSS has expressed concern about this informal system (*UK Press Gazette* 9 November 1992), complaining that it has not restrained some local newspapers sufficiently to prevent 'jigsaw identification'. This is where the putting together of details reported in one medium with those from another allows the audience to infer an identity, as happened in one of the cases discussed in Chapter 5 below.

Provisions in the Children Act 1989 allow reporters to be excluded from family proceedings or 'if he *is* allowed to remain he faces ... restrictions which will make it difficult for him to file a meaningful story' (Welsh and Greenwood 1992: 38; emphasis in original). Only very limited material can be published about parents or guardians bringing wardship proceedings before a judge in chambers, resulting in, according to Welsh and Greenwood (1992: 39), 'a danger to newspapers in publishing what is seen as a parent's struggle to retain control of a child'. Local authorities or others can also seek an injunction to prevent any reporting of family proceedings in the magistrates court or of cases relating to children heard in judge's chambers (Welsh and Greenwood 1992: 40).

The law also provides anonymity for children, women, and (since 1992) men who have been subjected to sexual attack (Welsh and Greenwood 1992: 51).

Newspapers challenged reporting restrictions in both the Rochdale child sex abuse events and the Frank Beck trial (both discussed below). For the *Daily Mail/Mail on Sunday* the use of injunctions became the subject of a continuing campaign (Walker 1992).

THE IMPACT OF THE NEWS MEDIA ON THE AUDIENCE

In his widely used text, McQuail wearily concludes: 'The entire study of mass communication is based on the premise that there are effects from the media, yet it seems to be the issue on which there is least certainty and least agreement' (1987: 251). This is not very surprising: we still know little about the physiology or psychology of perception and cognition, or of the link between self and society. Even if there were general agreement that empirical determination of media effects were possible, the fundamental methodological problems of the social sciences are raised in an unusually vivid form: what would have been the outcome in the absence of the media message under study? Many methodologists and media specialists would anyway argue that these are not simple empirical questions but, being in the political and philosophical arena, are essentially contested.

Nor is the debate over media effects clarified by its being a meeting point of different academic traditions with very different ideas about canons of argument, evidence and proof. McQuail provides a very useful review (1987: Chapter 9) demonstrating the dominance of the experimental psychology paradigm in media effects research from its inception alongside developing mass media at the beginning of the twentieth century. For several decades these new media were imputed with enormous power, linked to their assumed impact on mass movements in the early years of the Soviet Union and in Nazi Germany. This rather mechanistic model was then overtaken by an account which attributed much greater diversity of response and autonomy to the audience, allowing for 'intervening effects from personal contact and social environment' (McQuail 1987: 253).

In the late 1960s and 1970s this style of work, criticized as disregarding social structure and historical context, was challenged by a wholly different perspective on media influenced by the humanistic Marxism of the European New Left. Significant British examples of this examination of the setting of news 'agendas' are the Glasgow University Media Group's series (1976; 1980; 1985) of fiercely attacked but highly influential studies of television news, and Hall et al.'s (1978) account of the mobilization of public support for 'law and order' policies by identifying and demonizing the mugger. Latterly this tradition has been debunked in its turn for having only the crudest of assumptions about media effects: that the media are as powerful as their owners and state paymasters assume, and that the audience is passive and incapable of any kind of criticism and contextualization.

In many ways parallel to the 'uses and gratifications' revision of psychologically derived media theory during the immediate post-war era, much of the assault on what is seen as the over-determined Marxian tradition has come from literary theory. Attention has shifted from the 'text' to the use made of it. Media users are attributed with considerable sophistication in understanding not only media forms and their intertextual allusions but also the interests they embody. For example, Frazer (1987) challenges McRobbie's (1982) unquestioned assumption that young women are profoundly influenced by the messages about gender and domesticity embodied in apparently lightweight comics. They are, Frazer says, able to understand and comment on the stories as a conventional form, produced by a commercial organization for profit.

How far are readers/viewers able to bring the same powers of deconstruction to a 'negotiated reading' of the news? Recent work has been preoccupied with television, with Morley (1986) and Philo (1990) trying to map how viewers' gender, class, biography, and regional background are brought to bear on their use, recall and understanding of what they have seen. In both studies a key finding – and confirmation of earlier research – is that viewers are most likely confidently to challenge the version of events presented either when they have firsthand knowledge of those events, or of a situation parallel to it, or when a trusted informant provides counter-evidence. In relation to the 1984–5 miners' strike, staff in a Glasgow solicitors' office rejected the notion that the picketing was mostly violent for interwoven reasons: the radical political tradition of the area, the view (from Scotland) of the BBC as pro-establishment, and that they had actually passed peaceful picket lines in the locality. The corollary is that, where people have no other source of what they regard as reliable evidence, the media have the potential to set the news agenda in terms of both topics and discursive framework – a very important consideration where the complex and largely hidden world of social work is concerned.

Given the fascination with television, little work seems recently to have been done on the impact of newspaper messages. The press itself is highly ambivalent on the matter, as events around the April 1992 UK general election demonstrated. A large section of the national press vociferously supported the Conservative cause, not only in editorials, features and cartoons, but also by what was widely criticized elsewhere in the news media as a breakdown of the illusory but often repeated convention that news and comment are distinct and should be separate. Yet when the Labour Party, bewildered by an unexpected defeat, accused the press of contributing to the débâcle, the papers angrily denied that they had been an influence, claiming instead that they merely enabled the electorate to make a judgement on the facts. It was even suggested that the newspapers were free to be partisan precisely because most people did not take them seriously as a source of news!

When surveyed, the UK public undoubtedly claims that television is its preferred source of actuality (see Worcester 1991 for example) and yet how much is remembered? A paper by Gunter (1992), reviewing a decade of research on television news understanding and recall, prompts the heretical thought that, if people are only recalling about 50 per cent of what they have seen, perhaps they are more influenced than they concede by newspaper agendas. This possibility is underscored by Gunter's report of his own earlier finding that high recall was affected by 'talking to people about news and claimed frequency of watching national news on television'. If people are interested in news, perhaps they are more likely to buy/read newspapers. The mass tabloids are specifically intended to be a topic of conversation at home, at work and at leisure. The broadsheets are expecting advertisers to support them because they are part of the political and policy process. Surely it would be as great a mistake to relegate the influence of the press to a post-modern ultra-relativist porridge, where nothing and everything is significant, as to accept uncritically the power which the capitalist proprietors surely hope that it possesses.

MAKING THE NEWS

What then is 'news'? Newsgatherers and news processors simultaneously hold two contradictory models. On the one hand, they define newsworthiness as an intrinsic quality of some events, so that learning to be a good journalist is learning to spot this category. On the other, they acknowledge the social and cultural conventions that, within technical and organizational imperatives, construct news. This is neatly, perhaps unintentionally, captured by Boyd in his how-to-do-it manual: 'for most news editors the selection of news is more an art than a science. Stories are weighed up by an instinctive process they would put down to *news sense*' (1990: 4; emphasis in original). Yet later on (1990: 362) 'hard news' is defined as 'information of importance about events of significance'. Typically of journalists writing about their own profession, the definitions partly acknowledge the social and political context, but assume a consensus about 'events of significance'.

Boyd's formulation of the newsworthy event includes proximity, relevance, immediacy, interest and drama, which reflects many aspects of Galtung and Ruge's (1965) classic study of what characteristics lead events to be included in a newspaper. They identified twelve factors, suggesting that the higher the 'score', the more likely is the event to be classified as news.

- The *frequency* of the event has to fit the medium (so only some events of the previous week would still be 'news' for a Sunday paper).
- It must reach a certain *amplitude* (the heavier the snow or the larger the robbery).
- Events cannot be too *ambiguous* (the media had great difficulty with competing accounts in the early stages of the Cleveland affair).
- The event must be *meaningful* in terms of being culturally relevant or proximate (even a big, violent bank raid in Belgium is unlikely to make the UK news).
- It must be *consonant*, even expected or predicted and, if unexpected, capable of being fitted into existing ways of understanding. In Galtung and Ruge's famous epigram: all 'news' is 'olds'. (All injured brides-to-be are determined to walk up the aisle.)
- Despite this, there must be an element of the *unexpected or rare*. (The party conference is highly orchestrated and yet the leader is not given a standing ovation; an example of a species thought to be extinct is found.)
- Once an event becomes news it will have *continuity*, though probably with declining importance.
- *Composition* also plays a part in selection. In all newspapers there is a mix of types of news: home and overseas, serious and light.

The study also suggests four dimensions related to the specific cultures of 'the north-western corner of the world': that newsworthy events must relate to *élite nations*, *élite people*, must be *personalized* and are most likely to be defined as news if they are *negative*. Galtung and Ruge attribute the focus on persons to a combination of idealist/individualist cultural values, ease of identification, as part of the 'élite concentration' and because of its fit with newsgathering routines. 'Negativity', they propose, more often fits other criteria like rarity and unambiguity.

Despite the narrow base of the original data, Galtung and Ruge's criteria have proved very durable and are still recognizable for UK national papers, although how the factors are operationalized depends upon the market being addressed. What the *Guardian* can treat as unambiguous may be a problem in the different presentational format of the *Daily Mirror*; cultural proximity is undoubtedly different for the *Sun* and *The Independent*.

Most of the dimensions also apply, with scaled-down amplitude, proximity, and élites, to the local press. For local papers, though, negativity does not seem to have the same importance. Local papers are full of 'good news'. This contrast between local and national media is under-explored and under-theorized. If the underlying mechanism is audience identification, is the key that locality provides an assumptive basis of shared interest?

Once an event is categorized as news, how is it treated? This, even more than the initial selection, will reflect the characteristics of particular newspapers. Chibnall (1977: 23ff.) has classified eight factors which form an 'implicit guide to the construction of news stories': immediacy; dramatization; personalization; simplification; titillation; conventionalism; structured access; novelty. (Of these, structured access is more to do with defining and verifying news – see below – than its treatment.) It is not that 'quality' papers disdain drama, personalization, or titillation, rather that their definition is different from that in the mass tabloids. Pages may be given over to the resignation of a leading member of the Labour shadow cabinet, thus personalizing policy issues in a way parallel to but different from the tabloids' distilling problems with the pound sterling as 'Major at War With Germans'. Do the luscious, aspirational fantasy food and drink sections in the broadsheets serve the same titillating purpose as 'Page Three' girls?

But it cannot be argued that the ideas expressed in all papers are therefore the same, even leaving aside explicit political alignment. The sales pitch of the mass tabloids is based on the interpenetration of immediacy, dramatization, personalization and titillation with simplification. Perhaps the strongest nexus is between the simplification entailed in mass tabloid format and personalization, which further enables easy identification of the reader with the topic in hand. (Interestingly, despite television news organizations' trying to define themselves by analogy with newspapers – ITN *News at Ten* as mid-market; BBC *Nine O'Clock News* as broadsheet – the format, of visuals plus a text that must be uncomplicated enough to be grasped at first hearing, produces outcomes much in common with the mass tabloids.)

Immediacy plus drama plus simplification produces an emphasis on events and persons, rather than structures and processes. The situation in Northern Ireland thus becomes a series of fragments about who was shot by whom and who has just walked out of peace talks. How this point was arrived at is relegated to occasional features, which are themselves rare in the mass tabloids and more likely to be highly idiosyncratic diatribes in the mid-market papers.

These imperatives of news construction are embedded not just in choice of topic but also in the writing of individual items. A story is supposed to follow the chain who? – what? – when? – where? – how?, and a good 'professional' piece of copy will be capable of being sub-edited from the bottom up without loss of sense. The overall format of text, pictures and headlines also contributes to this historical foreshortening. Headlines, particularly in the mass tabloids, are in the present tense or are even verbless strings of nouns as 'Britons in crash horror'.

This said, the *Daily Mirror* on its best form can produce clarity without oversimplification, for example in a question-and-answer format article on the Salman Rushdie controversy. Many social work issues are complex personal scenarios, played out in a mystifying statutory frame-work, hedged about with political conflict and issues of confidentiality. Nevertheless, they could be amenable to this approach, for example: is imprisonment a deterrent to offending; are children always better off with their natural parents; what is the meaning of 'care in the community'? But no newspaper will devote resources to such a project unless the topic is thought to be interesting to their readers and the answers produced are going to fit into the paper's political agenda. Does the *Daily Express* actually want to establish that prison is counter-productive? Getting social work a 'better press' is not simply a matter of improved mutual understanding.

The focus on the here-and-now and on the individual may follow on from news routines and formats but it also has a powerful ideological effect. If structure and processes are not manifest they are less likely to be discussed, and if not discussed will not be challenged.

One of the many paradoxes of newsgathering and news processing is that 'news' connotes unexpectedness and yet a high proportion of what appears in news media is predictable. Were it not, it would be impossible to produce a paper of restricted size and format to a rigid daily schedule. News organizations are in permanent tension between boredom and drama, routine and chaos, an ideology of freebooting individualism and rigid hierarchic bureaucratic controls. Newspapers set out to be reassuringly familiar. Each has a distinctive style of typography, mode of address, field of news covered, and order of contents. All these are altered either by stealth or with considerable misgiving. Snow (1994) comments on the 'ontological security' provided by this predictable and routine quality. Arguably it increases the ideological impact of the medium's whole agenda, even if individual items are ignored, forgotten or subject to criticism.

In a daily newspaper the day starts with an editorial meeting to plan that day's edition. What to cover and its treatment will depend on the newspaper's position in the market and its editorial policies. While the broadsheets will devote considerable space to a party conference, a mass tabloid will only highlight the more dramatic episodes. A controversy over education may get extensive coverage in both the *Guardian* and the *Daily Mail*, but with very different inflection.

Predictability of news is vital to managing the enterprise, and is achieved in a range of ways. Even unexpected events may provide 'continuing news' with short-term predictability: an unforecast blizzard can yield follow-up stories/pictures about its impact on London's business life, isolated farms, etc. The crucial trade-off is how long interest value can be sustained. If major resources have been deployed – staff with their expenses or even cash payments to a source – there is an obvious incentive to find more 'angles'.

Many events are regular, especially in the state/political arena: the budget; the state opening of parliament. Many other formal public events are known in advance, like the start of a high-profile trial, the French referendum on the Maastricht Treaty, royal visits. This will be obvious to the readers, if they pause to reflect. What is less obvious is that many one-off events are also put into media organization's diaries well in advance. The main trade paper, *UK Press Gazette*, has a back page 'Gazetteer' each week, itself supplied by a specialist agency. Political, royal and sporting fixtures are prominent but the list includes, for example, launches of charity campaigns. Parallel processes will take place in local papers. Much of the news content of the paper will consist of these predicable events and stories picked up from other media – which are constantly and minutely scrutinized – leaving some slack for the truly unexpected.

A distinction is sometimes made between 'originating' and 'developing' news. The reality is that most newsgathering is in the latter category. 'Originating' news ranges from individual journalists pursuing ideas of their own to ambitious 'investigative reporting', which may lead to the longed-for but largely mythic 'exclusive'. Originality is expensive, one way or another. The famous pictures of the Duchess of York on holiday in Provence, which provided the *Daily Mirror* with a classic scoop, were obtained from a freelance photographer at a high price. 'Investigative reporting' is the closest that news media staff come to what is meant by 'research' in the wider society: starting out with an idea without being wholly sure where it will lead and whether the outcome will be worth the effort. For this reason, media organizations are, in reality, very cautious about it. Tying up staff in something that may go nowhere is a much higher risk than, say, sending a member of political staff to the Labour Party conference, which is bound to produce at least some news items and probably features too. As Soothill and Walby (1991) comment, crime is the only area in which the mass tabloids routinely undertake investigative work, often providing large amounts of material about the victim, the offence, the accused and a 'cascade' of detail about associated people at the end of a high-profile trial. The *Financial Times* devoted a team of staff over months to piece together the intricacies of Robert Maxwell's financial activities. Having produced dramatic revelations (*Financial Times* 6 November 1991) shortly before his death, their work has continued as his labyrinthine affairs are further revealed.

For most day-to-day purposes 'research' is a much more limited activity. Apart from the distinction between news and comment, journalists also separate 'hard' and 'soft' news. Boyd's definition of hard news is widely held, confident – and a tautology (1990: 362; see also Tuchman 1978: 48). In practice this philosophical quagmire is side-stepped by treating hard news as requiring some sort of proof. If it is hard news, rather than soft news or 'comment', then the conventions of objectivity must be followed. These are rarely related to 'reality' but are rather what Tuchman has called 'strategic ritual': the setting of one truth claim against another. Faced with a Greenpeace allegation that toxic waste is being illegally dumped at sea, the journalist will seek an authoritative source to comment, presumably to deny it. Alternatively, further sources may be used as confirmation, or the story reported but distancing words like 'claim' or 'allege' used. Inverted commas are often used to make clear what remains unproven: 'COP HELD OVER WIFE'S "FAKE CRASH DEATH"' (*Daily Mirror* 5 January 1993). Here the *Mirror* is protecting itself against contempt of court. They are also used to distance the paper from a point of view: 'POLL TAX CASH CUTS "LED TO TODDLER'S DEATH"' headed the *Sun*'s (21 June 1990) account of the Stephanie Fox inquiry report.

'Standing a story up' consists of getting enough credible informants to confirm it, or otherwise. Ericson *et al.* (1987: 173ff.) provide a detailed example of this. A Toronto local television journalist is sent to follow up a press clipping about a 'harbour crime wave'. She approaches the police, victims of theft, marina staff, and even passers-by, to try to substantiate the story, without success. While she is convinced that she has reliably established that there is no story, the editor who assigned her asks her to continue to try. 'Later the reporter commented about the fact that it was Monday, a slow news day because it follows the weekend when there is "no news"' (Ericson *et al.* 1987: 174). This instance also nicely illustrates that 'hard news', far from being a self-evident reality, is highly elastic, depending upon organizational context and competing events.

Tellingly, Boyd (1990) does not define 'soft news', presumably because he does not think it is what the business is about. In reality newspapers are full of it, whether amusing snippets or more substantial 'human interest', 'background' or 'colour' stories of the kind that will be prepared about, say, the victim's grieving family during a murder trial, for publication at its conclusion. Both content and process lack the macho associations that are so much a part of the ideology of newspaper journalism, but they are a vital part of the news agenda, particularly per-haps because voices are unchallenged. In a soft news item the foster mother's version of her 'heartbreak' because of the actions of the local social services will not be 'balanced' by a reply from the department. If she had spoken at a news conference, the offsetting account, if available, might well have been thought necessary.

How, then, to identify sources to stand a story up? Cuttings files, jealously guarded contact books and sources occupying official positions in formal structures will be invoked. The sophistication of these methods will depend upon whether the reporter is a specialist or a general reporter and whether the news relates to a regular 'newsbeat', like police or the courts, where even a junior reporter can quickly access standard sources of information. Much of state social work does not fall into this category, neither being on regular local newsbeats, nor having specialist corres-pondents in all national papers – even the broadsheets. Newsworthy events in local authority social services or probation may well be either covered by a generalist with little knowledge of the (ever-changing) statutory framework and current professional preoccupations, or refracted through the lens of crime news or political news, as Golding and Middleton (1982) observed in their analysis of social security in the news. Treacher (*Local Government Chronicle* 22 July 1988) also comments, in relation to the Cleveland events: 'many reporters were unaware of terms used by social services and the law'.

Whether the newsgatherer is a general reporter or heavyweight specialist on a broadsheet paper, the conventions by which stories are substantiated have three crucial consequences: old paradigms are reproduced; those with formal positions of influence will more often have their point of view given credence; and the tendency to reduce all issues to a binary opposition of for/against or praise/blame or hero/villain will be amplified. The political/ideological consequences of this are discussed in greater detail below.

If it not obvious from a casual reading of a newspaper how high a proportion of the items are pre-planned, it is even less obvious that much of the material is not gathered by the paper's own staff at all. News agencies have long been a source of foreign news and pictures (and may be almost the only source for mass tabloids, who do not direct their spending to foreign affairs). In the past many papers credited their use with a tag: Reuters, Agence France Presse, etc. This is no longer so, perhaps indicating a reluctance to admit to the extent to which they are relied upon. Within the UK, agencies provide national news and pictures for both national and local/regional papers and a plethora of local agencies provide local news/pictures for local and national media. The use of agencies for features and regular items like weather forecasts is also developing, partly as a result of newspapers driving to cut costs by reducing the number of their directly employed staff. National news-papers also use 'stringers', often working for local media, who will regularly supply stories on a freelance basis, some of which may get taken up. Another dimension of this process has been the further increase in the use of wholly freelance contributors and 'casual' staff employed for a shift at a time, both of whom are self-employed, have no security of employment and therefore have even less scope to resist editorial policy and pressures than 'permanent' staff in an industry renowned for its insecurity and brutal labour relations.

Close reading of the press also reveals the extent to which stories are simply lifted from other media, without acknowledgement: specialist journals to Sundays; weekend broadcasting and Sundays to weekday broadsheets; broadsheets to tabloids. On those occasions when a large number of newspapers are working simultaneously on a story, whether planned for or not, there is – apart from the rare exclusive – much sharing of information and ideas. Both staff in the field and editorial staff are desperate to have all the news that their immediate competitors have, producing a 'pack mentality' in both what is covered and how. The resulting similarity of coverage is then cited by journalists as evidence for the self-evidence of 'news' as a discrete category of events. It is better understood as the intersubjectivity of a highly introspective occupational group.

Local free papers exist by having an editorial staff ranging from small to tiny. Most of their 'news' is 'placed news' that is, supplied by the source of the news. Some of this is hardly distinguishable from advertising; indeed there is a new form known as 'advertorial' where copy set out in the same visual style as the rest of the newspaper is supplied by the subject of the news or an agency. Although paid-for local papers and national news media strike very disdainful attitudes about uncritical reproduction of such 'placed' news, the practice is not limited to free papers. Major local paid-for papers may produce features extolling the virtues of cosy village pubs. Were the pubs chosen after exhaustive and disinterested research? What is the relationship with the department store that seems to have supplied all the season's 'new, fresh, fashion look'? What about local radio using a ready-prepared tape, in the form of a news item, about British Telecom's latest technical achievements? It is not just local freesheets that use placed news thankfully because it saves on editorial costs: the practice is very pervasive, its boundary hard to define, and the news managers extend all the way from your local replacement window manufacturers to Downing Street.

This grey area where journalism meets advertising and PR is not new. Fashion, motoring and sports journalism have long been defined as lacking status within the profession because of perceived over-dependence on sources (Tunstall 1971). That sports writers are very highly paid, and crucial to the success of the paper in the case of the mass tabloids, is a further irony of journalism's professional ideology. It is given another twist by the wholesale reproduction of company PR on the business pages of broadsheets of every persuasion. The arts pages of the broadsheets are also effectively acting as publicity for commercial products in the form of books, recorded music, art galleries and the commercial theatre.

Not that competition for access to the media is limited to politicians and for-profit enterprises. One of the consistent policies of Tory governments since 1979 has been to impose, as far as possible, market-style behaviour on social institutions which are not run for profit. One aspect of this, described vividly in respect of the players in the criminal justice field by Schlesinger et al. (1991), is the need to justify the allocation of public funds by the extra-parliamentary means of media exposure. Thus the police co-operate with the proliferating television series dramatizing crime, the prison service allows television crews to make 'warts and all' documentaries displaying the squalor in gaols to try and increase cash for rebuilding, and even HM Customs and Excise tries to establish that it is friendly and exciting, not just the VATman.

News management, whether by public agencies or by commercial and industrial firms, is now much more sophisticated than simply the issuing of news releases, although these continue to multiply. Events of a visual kind have to be staged, and as dramatically as possible. Although this is primarily in response to television's need for pictures, events have a useful concreteness for print journalism too. Reports by pressure groups are no longer published and sent to news organizations with a handy summary, they are 'launched'. Even academic conferences and universities issue news releases – and increasingly seem to get coverage.

Revealing the use of placed news ranges from frank acknowledgement to near-dishonesty. 'Psychiatric services are failing to provide women with the help they need, emphasising drugs or other treatments rather than counselling and social support, a report from the mental health charity MIND says today' (*Guardian* 28 September 1992) is a model of transparency, alongside an item which is similarly open about its basis on a Vegetarian Society staged event. But what of a *Daily Mail* (12 April 1991) article 'Lenient probation officers may end up in court'? Did the bylined Home Affairs Correspondent doorstep the Home Office to find out? It is much more likely that 'the Home Office said yesterday' is code for an official news release about the Criminal Justice Bill (now 1991 Act). 'Revealed' is another popular way of indicating information gained either from a news conference or even simply written up from material supplied directly to the news organization.

When journalists give accounts of their own work, the emphasis is always a romanticized vision of buccaneering newsgathering, which reaches its apotheosis in the war or foreign correspondent under fire. In the newspaper as a marketable product, however, that kind of 'news' plays a very small part, as we have seen. Nevertheless, journalists are still going out to cover events, sometimes even against the wishes of the participants. What happens to the material they collect? Few journalists can expect their news copy to appear virtually unchanged in the paper; this is the prerogative of star foreign correspondents and political writers. Even specialists may find their articles rejected or edited to fit within space and priorities. General reporters may have their work virtually rewritten by sub-editors, the unseen but crucial mediators in the news process.

On a morning daily paper, sub-editors and other editorial staff will work evenings/nights, thus leading an even more hermetic existence than other journalists. It is they who ensure that the paper's editorial policies of style and content are consistently applied.

The newspaper as a whole consists of news, features, editorials, pictures and advertisements presented in the paper's distinctive idiom. Media research has, so far, been less successful in evaluating this overall package than in discussing the surface or near-surface of news texts and their headlines. That 'a picture is worth a thousand words', though it has become a cliché of news production, is still thought to be true, although both media analysts and practitioners have difficulty in explaining why. In Evans's *Pictures on a Page* (1978) he grapples with the mystery of the continuing impact of black-and-white still photographs in an age of colour television. He concludes that they serve better as symbols. A vivid example of this is the photograph of Winston Silcott who was tried and sentenced for the murder of a policeman, and subsequently cleared on appeal. Although an apparently simple full-length, face-on portrait, the circumstances in which it was taken produced an image of Winston Silcott as not only black but animalistic. This was ruthlessly exploited by those papers whose agendas on both race and 'law and order' had increased the pressure on the police for results at any price. (Hall (1981) and Hartley (1982) also discuss the analysis of newspaper photographs, drawing on semiotic concepts, the potential of which remains largely unrealized in the analysis of news media.)

The 'voice' of a newspaper is extremely complex: the popular style of the mass tabloids requires at least as much skill to achieve with consistent success as the more obvious elegance of *The Independent*. Fowler (1991) draws attention to the sheer range of linguistic devices used by the *Sun* – not just the obvious puns, alliteration and rhyming:

> Interestingly, the *Sun* indulges in 'poetic' structures in places where it is being at its most outrageous about politics or sex. Cues are fore-grounded to the point of self-parody. Deplorable values are openly displayed, pointedly highlighted; even a critical reader can be disarmed by pleasure in the awfulness of the discourse.
>
> (Fowler 1991: 45)

Quite.

Some of the intended effects of newspaper language are not hard to identify; the crude racism of the *Sun*'s references to 'Frogs' and 'Krauts' and to Arabs as 'pigs'; policy decisions that transform 'terrorists' through 'guerillas' to 'army' (or vice versa); the pervasive use of military language not only for policing but, for example, for the tightening of social security regulations. Only amateur scepticism is needed to see where the *Daily Express* (4 May 1992) is coming from: 'Parents who smack their children could soon be hauled before the courts on a criminal charge. But the proposal divided the nation last night when a Tory MP said the suggestion was "absolutely absurd"'. Are criminals 'hauled' before the courts?

Fowler (1991) applies sophisticated techniques of linguistic analysis to the UK press, demonstrating some of the less obvious ways that language is used to construct 'us'/'them', reassuring/threatening, order/ instability. I shall take only three examples from a book that contains true 'revelations'.

- The use of familiar and conversational forms in written text. Commenting on government policy in the style 'Come off it, mate' implies that the paper is on the same wavelength as its readership (being on informal terms), is cheekily not overawed by authority, and yet can speak authoritatively on behalf of its mass public – and therefore should be heard in a liberal democracy. Many of the *Sun*'s colloquialisms are oddly out of date: 'toffs', 'boffins'. In some cases this seems to encode the out-of-dateness of the subject; in others historical continuity and nationhood is being invoked as in calling Gulf War soldiers, many of whom would have been born after 1970, 'desert rats'. The North African battle with Rommel's army took place in 1942.
- The deployment of 'we', 'you' and 'they' forms does not always catch attention, but is very important in classifying 'them', the pivot on which much news turns. Fowler describes it as part of 'consensus building'. A set of 'positive legitimating values' is contrasted with 'negative illegitimate values' in binary opposition, for example, self-reliance versus dependency. Positive terms are then linked with political objectives and 'we' are represented as endorsing them. If trade union action is extremism, we must be against it, because we are moderate. If health service cuts are gains in efficiency then we must be in favour, because only 'they' advocate waste (Fowler 1991: 51–2, quoting Chibnall 1977: 21–2). Since social work is often operating on the deviancy boundary it is particularly open to this type of reinforcement of its marginality.
- Fowler also sets out the ways in which participants in the news can be rendered active or passive and, by implication, responsibility/power heightened or modified. Compare 'PC SHOT BOY FROM 9 INCHES' with 'Robber's son, five, killed in his bed' and 'BOY WAS SHOT BY PC FROM 9 INCHES' (Fowler 1991: 77–8). In one of his extended examples Fowler (1991: 125–34) unpicks a feature (intended to be sympathetic) on the effect of health service shortages on patients. They are categorized by age or illness or length of wait, so that they are conveyed as powerless 'experiencers' who 'are rarely agents of actions and these are usually actions that affect only the patient him-/herself'. The parallels with the coverage of elderly people (when covered at all, see Chapter 4) and people with disabilities is obvious (and the subject of pressure group action).

Who determines the paper's 'voice' and alignment? Editors still wish to claim this capacity but, as far as many of the UK national papers are concerned, it is increasingly apparent that if they have room for manoeuvre it is because they have been appointed precisely because they share the proprietor's perspective (Evans 1983; Hollingsworth 1985). Rupert Murdoch is famously quoted as 'not having come all this way not to interfere' (Hollingsworth 1985: 18) but 'it would be unfair to depict [him] as the biggest bogeyman of all. They are all at it,' writes Bevins (1990) as he mounts a scathing attack on the willingness of editors to bow to proprietors and journalists to editors, suggesting that all the pressures are towards accepting editorial policy on what is covered and how. He further suggests, however, that in turn proprietors are vulnerable to political pressure.

PROFESSIONAL IDEOLOGY AND POWER

All occupations have a shared system of beliefs. In the case of journalism it is very highly developed, frequently articulated, and replete with myth. The remoteness of this myth from the reality of the contemporary workplace is itself vital to understanding both the daily work of the press and its place in the political and social order.

Journalists seem to be compulsive biographers and autobiographers. A repeated theme of these accounts is the 'self-made' person – usually male. This is not entirely illusory: despite the growth of graduate-entry schemes, it is still possible to repeat the experience of many currently practising journalists, who started on a local paper in their mid-teens straight from school. Derek Jameson (former editor of the *Daily Express*, *Daily Star*, and *News of the World*) writes (1989; 1990) vividly of his childhood poverty; Kelvin MacKenzie (editor of the *Sun* during its outrageous 1980s era) is said to fudge the fact that he left a good school with some formal qualifications (Chippindale and Horrie 1990).

These biographies, whether books or articles in the trade papers, stress hard living: long hours, drinking, smoking, explosive leisure pursuits – really being one of the lads. And that includes many of the women who have achieved enough seniority to be profiled.

Newsgathering is highly competitive: trying to get copy back to the paper before other media do; competing to get a piece in the paper at all. The resulting inability to work in a team was commented upon by psychiatrists attached to the forces during the Falklands campaign (Morrison and Tumber 1988). They predicted that it would result in additional stress under combat conditions, correctly in a number of instances. Rather than increasing the fabled self-reliance, this competition actually engenders a high degree of insecurity and need for praise and reassurance (also observed with puzzlement by the military during the Falklands campaign). As recession has taken its toll of jobs and of union recognition and speeded up the casualization of the workforce, competition has further intensified. Presumably this has made the imposition of managerial control still easier, especially since the dispersal of national newspaper offices all over London has made even informal alliances of staff hard to create.

Collectivism, then, never very strong among journalists, has been even further displaced by the 'rooted and consistent individualism' reported by Golding and Middleton (1982: 142) in their study of social security/social work news. They go on to suggest that this anti-bureaucratic, anti-claiming, anti-'dependency culture' rhetoric is an important element in understanding the reporting of social work news, by making even liberally inclined journalists unable to comprehend the systemic basis of poverty and disadvantage: '"I have never been a claimant . . . It would mean I had no initiative to find a job . . . The welfare state is outside the experience of most journalists"' (Golding and Middleton 1982: 143). The speaker is Melanie Phillips, who still writes for the *Guardian* and may well have come to a different view, but the reductionist perspective lives on. In a 1992 *60 Minutes* television documentary a woman journalist for *Mail on Sunday* remarks that 'a lot of iffy people' work with child sex abuse. In other words, that, far from being inscribed in the social construction of gender relations and family life, child sex abuse is not even a societal problem; it may not even be real at all, just the pre-occupation of a group of pathological people.

Alongside individualism in the occupational ideology, goes an idea of 'professionalism'. This includes the technical skills, discussed above, of gathering the material needed, standing it up and producing copy in a form that is worth printing and needs little sub-editing. It also includes an element of inauthenticity which serves to obscure the contradiction between the profession's exaggerated belief in personal autonomy and the actuality of tight schedules, declining resources and domineering management. The 'professional' can produce the goods even if s/he does not share the values embodied. Derek Jameson (1989; 1990) describes how he managed to edit the (very) Tory *Daily Express* while holding socialist personal beliefs. Professionals can also produce a story or a new 'angle' from very little when the situation demands. Thus the Princess of Wales fanning herself on an otherwise utterly uneventful royal tour becomes 'Heat Hell'.

This dimension of professional skill illustrates the complex attitude to 'reality' already discussed. Accepting the full extent to which 'news' is not a discrete phenomenon but is, rather, entirely socially constructed would have dramatic consequences. All the conventions about truth and verification would be undermined:

> like the source bureaucracies they report on, journalists must publicly traffic the 'as if' world of procedural propriety to sustain their sense of legitimacy ... Thus objectivity, fairness and balance serve as public-culture legitimation for journalistic practices. This implanting helps to explain the central place of investigative reporting both in the working culture of journalists and the public mythology about journalism. The belief is created both within the craft and publicly that 'real reporting' consists of extensive investigation and profound discovery using multiple sources and methods and arriving at the truth. Journalists internalize this 'as if' world even in the face of the fact that it could not be farther from the truth of what their work actually consists of.
>
> (Ericson *et al.* 1987: 358)

No doubt this is why media professionals react so angrily to social scientists' interest in the 'making' of news: if you believe that news is 'objective facts', then there is little difference between 'making' and 'faking' (Schudson 1989).

The series by Ericson and his colleagues (1987; 1989; 1991) is important for a number of reasons. First, it is a recent study of news organizations' working practices (in newspapers and television in Toronto) at a time when media studies seem in danger of a total pre-occupation with transnational business configurations and the geopolitics of communications. Second, it provides a wealth of detail about how news is actually produced (demonstrating the extent, for example, that television's demand for visuals results in the staging and restaging of events). Third, and most importantly, it is a robust defence of a pluralist model of media in the social structure, very much in the North American tradition, and will serve to open a discussion of the major theoretical cleavages in media theory over the relationship of sources to the power structure.

Why the preoccupation with sources? It relates to the pivotal importance of 'standing up' or verifying a story, for which journalists turn to reliable sources. 'Reliability' comes more often than journalists concede from occupying a position in a formal organization and these too have a hierarchy: state or public agencies above voluntary; big pressure groups above small ('Beware of unrepresentative groups with only a handful of members' (Boyd 1990: 17)); small pressure groups above the unaffiliated. Some sources are so credible that their statements will be accepted as news without verification – although they might be challenged in the form of feature or comment. If a government news release says new benefits regulations will target those in need more effectively, those news media that support the party in power are likely to frame the story in those terms, with more or less enthusiasm. Dissenting voices may be quoted to show 'balance' or, in the case of broadcast news, to fulfil the statutory requirement to be impartial but 'arguments against a primary definition are forced to insert themselves into *its* definition of "what is at issue"' (Hall *et al.* 1978: 68; emphasis in original). Even the dissent is likely to be sought from an organized forum like the Child Poverty Action Group. Consider the alternative: seeking a range of claimants, calculating the effect of the changes on them, obtaining their opinion of the new situation and framing the whole story as 'Government benefit changes: complicated package with very variable outcomes'. This may be nearer the 'truth' but, having used considerable resources in its production, it does not fit the imperatives of a news item in many daily papers – even if they are opposed to the party in power. Such coverage is consigned to features, documentaries, specialist journals and fringe newspapers.

Ericson *et al.* (1987; 1989; 1991) conceive of the news media as playing a crucial role in the negotiation of the boundaries of deviance, and as a corollary, the mechanisms of control in a 'knowledge society'. In this respect they are reiterating on the grand scale the views of many local journalists as described by Franklin and Parton (1991): that publishing the details of even minor court appearances is a vital part of the maintenance of social order. Not that Ericson and colleagues are guilty of vulgar pluralism. They do not model society as a kind of Elysian baseball game, where all players are equally skilled and follow the rules with only minor and quickly resolved disputes. On the contrary, much of their study is taken up with describing the handling of conflict: between editors and journalists, and news organizations and sources, whether trying to gain media coverage or keep it out. In their second volume (1989) they contrast the capacity of the court system – as a vital source – to dictate terms on access to the media (as do most private organizations, most of the time) with the increasingly symbiotic relationship between media, particularly the more populist, and the police. Ericson and colleagues accept and demonstrate that some persons and organizations are further up the 'hierarchy of credibility' (in Becker's (1967) classic phrase) than others, and that both individuals and organizations will pursue their own interests, but the hierarchy itself does not systematically and inevitably embody the interests of one section of society at the expense of others. The power structures of society have 'legitimacy', being in place and continuing by the consent of the majority in a democratic system. More analogous to a real baseball game in fact: conflictful but ultimately rule-bound.

In a UK context, Schlesinger *et al.* (1991) explore some of the same issues in their examination of the ways in which social control agencies compete for media attention as a means of defending or increasing their resources. Apart from their fascinating data on, for example, the relationship between the police, *Crimewatch*, and the audience, they are taking a theoretical position questioning what they see as the mono-polization of recent UK media research by the 'dominant ideology thesis', which:

> Using either a neo-Gramscian theory of 'hegemony' or a 'propaganda' model' [argues] that the power of politically and economically dominant groups in the society defines the parameters of debate, ensures the privileged reproduction of their discourse, and, by extension, largely determines the contours of the dominant ideology – of what is socially thinkable.

> (Schlesinger *et al.* 1991)

Schlesinger and colleagues go on to argue that within the 'policy arena' it is not the case that some players are able, unopposed, to define the issues and the terms in which they should be debated. On the contrary, there is constant struggle to be heard, involving not just government and departments of state, and state-funded agencies such as the prison and probation service, but other players like professional associations, campaigning pressure groups and voluntary agencies. They assert that the 'dominant ideology' thesis rests upon a tautological definition in which the capacity to be 'primary definer' of an issue derives a priori from institutionalized power, embodied in the state, which must axiomatically represent the dominant class interest. Schlesinger and his colleagues nevertheless have difficulty breaking free from this. They concede that the 'apparatuses of state' like the Home Office and the Metropolitan Police occupy the 'most advantageous locations' in the policy arena. They then go on to describe how 'more radical groups like Women in Prison' will achieve change by unpublicized negotiation, or threat of publicity. On occasion these groups may even be fed information to fuel a controversy in which one state agency is in dispute with another. While such manoeuvres certainly do not conform with a highly mechanistic model of the complete control of the news media by sources, neither do they demonstrate a much more open power structure. 'Primary definition' is not, after all, claimed to be 'only definition'.

The terms 'primary' and 'secondary definers' were refined by Hall and colleagues (1978) in their influential study of UK media treatment of mugging in the 1970s, which provides a classic example of writing in the 'dominant ideology paradigm'. Crude conspiracy theory is specifically rejected: 'the "reproduction of the dominant ideologies" . . . is the product of a set of *structural imperatives*, not of an open conspiracy with those in powerful positions'. These 'structural imperatives' include:

> two aspects of news production – the practical pressures of constantly working against the clock and the professional demands of impartiality and objectivity – [which] combine to produce a systematically structured *over-accessing* to the media of those in powerful and privileged social positions. The media thus tend . . . to reproduce symbolically the existing structure of power in society's institutional order.
>
> (Hall *et al.* 1978: 58; emphases in original)

THE IDEA OF THE 'MORAL PANIC'

'Moral panic' is one of the concepts developed in sociology that has passed into everyday discourse. In doing so, some of the complexities of the idea have been lost: a moral panic is not a 'lot of fuss about nothing'. Considering the provenance of the concept and its complexities is particularly important for the understanding of news about social work, as the idea was developed and elaborated in relation to criminal justice issues, has been used in relation to child abuse and in the UK urban disorders of 1981 and 1985, and is in dispute between analysts of the societal response to AIDS.

Stan Cohen's book *Folk Devils and Moral Panics* first appeared in 1972. Using the 'mods and rockers' phenomenon of 1964 onwards, it elaborates an interactionist model of deviance in which the news media take a central part. Cohen describes a cycle of phases, derived from the study of natural disasters: warning; impact; inventory; reaction. In the mods and rockers panic the initial events were minor skirmishes at Clacton on the bleak Easter Sunday of 1964. Monday being a 'slow news day' (see the Toronto marina saga above), these got the big treatment: 'Wild Ones Invade Seaside – 97 arrests' (*Daily Mirror* cited in Cohen 1973: 30). The 'inventory' stage, characterized by 'exaggeration' and 'distortion', is the drawing together of supposed characteristics which will eventually become shorthanded into a 'symbolization' and used in 'prediction'. When newspapers talked of 'another Clacton' they mobilized a whole array of ideas about violent gangs of newly affluent youngsters with no respect for authority rampaging down from London to inflict expensive damage on seaside resorts. As Cohen establishes, almost none of the supposed characteristics bore much relation to reality. But they provided a good peg for predictable news coverage, including pictures of empty beaches: 'Hastings – Without Them' (*Daily Mirror* on the Whitsun holiday 1965, cited in Cohen 1973: 39).

During the 'reaction' phase, media and control culture engage in debate about causes and there will be 'sensitization' to events that might not normally have passed the news threshold, as in the national newspaper reporting of 'normal' attacks by pet dogs during the 'dangerous dogs' furore. In this phase, crucially, the criminal justice system may well be involved, with the public rituals of exemplary sentences, portentous speeches from the bench, and demonization of offenders. Cohen points out that many of the alleged offences at Clacton and parallel episodes were very much in the area of police definition and discretion, like 'breach of the peace', making the amplification of the whole affair hard to resist. At this stage of a panic it will become a platform for parliamentary and pressure group politics, calling for stiffer sentences, less violence on television, more effective registration of dogs or whatever. If Cohen were writing today he might have laid even more emphasis on commercial exploitation: not just 'Are You a Mod?' quizzes in the mass tabloids, but all the lifestyle consumables to go with it.

Unlike the natural disaster, the moral panic has an embedded circularity, particularly following from the prediction aspect of the reaction phase. This message has been understood by social control agencies in, for example, the calls for the news media not to give routine coverage to behaviour on the terraces and outside the ground at football matches.

A key part of Cohen's argument is that the events he describes were neither unusual nor serious. Their explosion into public attention was largely by chance, given the lack of competing news. Cohen is not, however, arguing that the panic was unimportant. On the contrary, he sees it as the symbolic expression of contemporary currents of profound social change awaiting some episode to throw them into focus. These changes centred on working-class affluence, in particular the dramatic relative increase in disposable income of young people and the challenge this posed to traditional structures of family- and age-related authority. The social parameters of normality and deviance were in flux, engendering a 'modern morality play in which good (the police and the courts) met evil (the aggressive delinquent). Like all morality plays ... there was little doubt about which side would win: the devil's place was known in advance' (Cohen 1973: 39).

Cohen's image of the morality play is very significant, invoking images of a less fragmented, pre-industrial, organic and integrated society. In other words Cohen appears to be making assumptions about fundamental social consensus in the same mode as Ericson *et al.* (1987; 1989; 1991) discussed earlier. For this he was extensively criticized and it is this which distinguishes his study from Hall *et al.*'s superficially comparable but theoretically diametrically opposed *Policing the Crisis* (1978).

Hall and his colleagues analyse the relationship between the news media in the treatment of 'mugging' in the early 1970s. As in the mods and rockers events there was extensive publicity to this new threat to public order: coverage of court cases, exemplary sentences, public pronouncements by police, judiciary, politicians and pressure groups, reflexively citing newspaper coverage to confirm the importance of the issue both for the public and within the control culture. The argument of the book is, however, in many ways opposite to Cohen's position: that 'mugging' was a term imported from the US (with all its connotations of rampant crime and urban racial disorder) and applied by the police to a range of offences, many of which were hardly violent (like pick-pocketing), had been always been with us, and were anyway not increasing significantly. (Arguably, this last assertion about the lack of reality of the phenomenon and, therefore, the artificiality of public concern is the pivot of the book's case. Surprisingly little space is given to substantiating it in a book otherwise weighed down with citation and allusion, a weakness seized upon by critics like Waddington (1986).)

The contention of *Policing the Crisis* is that, faced with a 'crisis of legitimation' – that is, the justification of its structures and power – the dominant class, through the apparatuses of state, needed to get public support behind increased powers and resources for overt social control. The focus on street crime, with its demonization of already marginal disadvantaged black young men, came from the police using their status as 'primary definers', and was eagerly taken up by some sections of the media as part of a theme – 'our violent society' (also discussed by Chibnall 1977).

The place of violence in this moral panic, according to Hall and colleagues, is central, as part of what they describe as the 'signification spiral' (1978: 223–7). This process, they suggest, consists of two sub-processes: convergence, and the concept of 'thresholds'. 'Convergence' is the bracketing of previously unrelated phenomena into a new phenomenon with an 'imputed common denominator'. Thus political demonstrations and street crime become 'mindless violence'. According to Hall *et al.* this bracketing together, instigated by the primary definers of the control culture, will then be taken up by news media, perhaps with relish, grouping news under dramatic logos ('The mugger menace' or similar) and inviting sympathetic experts to write features. Even the broadcasters, statutorily bound not to editorialize, may adopt the convergence, as Glasgow University Media Group (1976) demonstrated in their account of television treatment of the economy and labour relations in the mid-1970s. A whole range of unrelated strikes, and even lock-outs, were swept together into single descriptive news items.

'Thresholds' are the boundaries of four concentric circles which Hall *et al.* use as a metaphor for levels of social control. At the centre is 'civilized society'. Then there is 'permissiveness', where activities like adultery are not approved but are not subject to legal sanctions either. The third ring, beyond legality, includes 'normal crime' and 'lesser' forms of 'violence' like 'violent demonstrations'. Beyond that is the 'extreme violence' of murder, treason, terrorism, etc. The argument of the study is that, since the state has the monopoly of legitimate violence, if activities can be categorized as beyond the legality boundary then they automatically become subject to state control. If something is not already a crime, establishing or reconceptualizing it as 'violent' has the same effect by putting it outside legitimate behaviour. (The media image of the picketing in the miners' strike of 1984–5 as characteristically rather than exceptionally violent is described in Philo (1990).) The corollary of this, of course, is that violence must itself be exceptional, which explains why claims that violence is pervasive in family life are so angrily resisted, especially in some sectors of the Conservative press.

In essence, then, the cycle of events described in both the Cohen and the Hall *et al.* studies is very similar, but their interpretation parts company over the issue of class interest. For Cohen the news media are an important component in a modern plural democracy, but are engaged in permanent dialogue with other interest groups. Drawing on the dominant ideology paradigm, Hall and his co-researchers are concerned to demonstrate how the state will inevitably – although rarely in an organized and intentional way – facilitate the interests of the ruling class. Since nearly all news media are either run for capitalist profit or effectively under state control, they will be forced into the position of 'secondary definers'. Even when it is radical and oppositional, social work is locked in an embrace with the control culture. The rest of this book will be about the triangular relationship between social work, the press and the state.

SUGGESTED FURTHER READING

Boyd, A. (1990) *Broadcast Journalism* (revised edition), Oxford: Heinemann.

Curran, J. and Seaton, J. (1991) *Responsibility Without Power: the Press and Broadcasting in Britain* (fourth edition), London: Routledge.

Ericson, R.V., Baranek, P.M. and Chan, J.B.L. (1987) *Visualizing Deviance*, Milton Keynes: Open University Press.

Fowler, R. (1991) *Language in the News*, London: Routledge.

Franklin, B. and Murphy, D. (1991) *What News? The Market, Politics and the Local Press*, London: Routledge.

Hartley, D. (1982) *Understanding News*, London: Methuen.

Negrine, R. (1989) *Politics and the Mass Media in Britain*, London: Routledge.

Philo, G. (1990) *Seeing and Believing: the Influence of Television*, London: Routledge.

Welsh, T. and Greenwood, W. (1992) *McNae's Essential Law for Journalists* (twelfth edition), London: Butterworths.

Part II

The case studies

Chapter 2

A child dies

Until the Cleveland events of 1987–8, the symbol of social work's 'bad press' was a sad list of children's names, connoting criminal trials for the killing of a child, perhaps followed by an official inquiry. The venom of some press comment in these cases, saturated with the assumption that social work intervention must have failed, seems to have led many in the profession to assume that any similar instance will inevitably produce the same kind of news coverage.

In this chapter the national daily press accounts of a number of cases between 1985 and 1991 will be scrutinized. The case of Tyra Henry is an illustration of a cluster of trials in the mid-1980s which received large-scale press treatment, much of it very hostile to social work. Later the same year the circumstances of the death of Charlene Salt, which could be seen as parallel in some respects to those surrounding Tyra Henry's, were the subject of more limited and muted coverage. The other case examples are of trials where national press reporting was low-key or even absent. By these, I hope to demonstrate that, even in the popular press, the vilification of social work is not an automatic reflex but is precipitated (even over-determined) by the presence or absence of a number of key variables of time, place, political regime, ethnicity, and news values.

While court proceedings are pending or taking place, news coverage is severely circumscribed: there can only be a description of the court-room events. Editorializing is limited to how much prominence is given to the case in terms of position in the paper, the aspects of the proceedings picked out in headlines, and whether pictures and other presentational devices to highlight the issue are used. These restraints end with the verdict: at that point overt judgements can be introduced through the news text, background 'colour' pieces like interviews with relatives, editorials and features.

THE TYRA HENRY CASE

In July 1985, Andrew Neil was tried at the Old Bailey for the murder of his daughter Tyra Henry, aged 21 months. The trial lasted four days; at its conclusion Neil, who had pleaded not guilty to murder, was sentenced to life imprisonment. Claudette Henry, Tyra Henry's mother was not charged with any offence, her evidence at the trial received heavy press coverage. Both Andrew Neil and Claudette Henry are African-Caribbean.

The *Guardian* gave the case prominent coverage on each day of the trial. The first day's proceedings were described on the front and back pages, with a small picture of the accused and a picture of Tyra Henry on p. 2. On day two, the trial was at the top of p. 2: 'Bite marks baby was under council care' (*Guardian* 24 July 1985). By day three the story was in the lower part of p. 3. The sentencing of Neil was the second lead on p. 1 (*Guardian* 26 July 1985), continued on the back page. Equal space was given in the report to the key events of the case and to the local political context. The judge's declaration that social workers were not at fault appears in the fourth paragraph, immediately followed by a statement from the vice-chairman of Lambeth Social Services that disciplinary action against staff was being contemplated.

The style of coverage is low-key to the point of dryness, both in tone and presentational style – almost in inverse relationship to the obvious local controversy. This emerged on the following day when the same named reporter who had covered the case 'reports on the rift between social workers and local authorities' (*Guardian* 27 July 1985). The prominent article (top of p. 3, with standfirst and photo of council leader) reports a demonstrative strike by staff in Lambeth against the proposed disciplinary measures resulting from an internal inquiry. (The strike ended when assurances were given that no such proceedings would be pursued until the outcome of the public inquiry. When it reported in December 1987 – see below – all disciplinary charges were dropped.) BASW is quoted, asserting that the politicization of local government was leading to local councillors' rejecting professional advice in the belief that it was insensitive to community needs. 'Balance' is built in by mentioning examples of both left- and right-wing councils and through the words of a 'senior officer': '"I do think professionals need to be challenged about what are appropriate values".' It is clear that ethnicity is at the centre of the Lambeth dispute; again the claims of both 'sides' are reported.

Coverage in the *Guardian* concluded on 29 July when an item on the lower half of p. 4 reported that a minister had asked for an 'immediate report' from Lambeth. The minister's apparent defence of professional over political judgements in child abuse cases is set in the context of NALGO/BASW complaints and the local political response. During the case and its immediate aftermath the *Guardian* made no editorial comment.

The first day of the trial was reported as the lead on p. 3 of the *Daily Telegraph*. The item was illustrated with a small photo of Andrew Neil. By day two, the story had moved up to occupy most of the news space on p. 2. Two stories were grouped with a photograph of Tyra Henry's mother arriving at the court. The third day of the trial was reported in a low-key item at the bottom of p. 2, but the verdict and sentence were given considerable prominence. 'LIFE SENTENCE FOR TYRA'S FATHER; Brother blinded in earlier incident' is the p. 1 lead, under the strapline 'Social services inquiry ordered' (*Daily Telegraph* 26 July 1985). The treatment also includes a secondary item: 'Row over who was to blame' and two pictures, the larger a neutral picture of Andrew Neil; below it is a picture of Tyra Henry in intensive care. (This is part of a larger picture given much prominence in some other papers earlier in the trial.) The 'row' story sets out the contrasting views of the judge and local politicians. It continues on the back page with a small picture of Janet Boateng, who is described as 'chairman of Lambeth's social service [*sic*] committee, and a well-known black rights campaigner. She is the wife of Mr Paul Boateng, chairman of the Greater London Council's police committee and Labour's prospective parliamentary candidate for Brent East' (*Daily Telegraph* 26 July 1985). The main focus is on the disputes in Lambeth over the policy document for use when working with black families, which is described as 'controversial' and is quoted. In the concluding paragraph the poverty of the area is mentioned and the deputy director of social services' statement calling for more resources is reported. A further item on p. 3, headed 'Tyra case workers accused of naivety', opens by drawing a parallel with the Jasmine Beckford case earlier the same year. The text is a neutral descriptive account of the internal inquiry report; it concludes with an observation about the difficulties facing social workers.

On 27 July the *Daily Telegraph* published a feature by June Lait (see Chapter 8) and alongside it a second leader highly critical of all parties involved. Social workers are 'soft-hearted social engineers' in a system that 'lurches from crisis to crisis'. The writer's accusation is that 'the ruling Labour group is accused of putting ideology before the welfare of children'. The piece concludes: 'if we are to have a social services system that takes away individual responsibility, the social workers should be spared from implementing the political theories of MRS BOATENG' (capitals in original – as for all proper names). The leader writer thus manages to elide legal responsibility for children in the council's care with the implicit yet completely unjustified suggestion that Mrs Boateng is personally responsible. The same motif appeared in the *Daily Express* coverage described below.

Daily Telegraph coverage continued with reports of the strike action and on 31 July the paper's third leader took up the charges and counter-charges flying between officers, unions and politicians in Lambeth. Two paragraphs in then-typical *Telegraph* style, complete with archaisms and circumlocutions, again castigate all in sight. Blaming central government would be 'neither fair nor accurate . . . but the Left is not overblessed with either of these virtues'. Then, in the last paragraph, a surprising turn, with an observation about the treatment of Andrew Neil and of a white man who had beaten his step-daughter to death and been sent to a probation hostel. There is a veiled but unmistakable criticism that the race of the defendant had affected the sentence.

The *Daily Express* gave the case prominent coverage from the first day, with pictures of the injuries to Tyra Henry on p. 1 and a report with pictures on p. 2. On day two the trial was reported on p. 10. The opening paragraph on 'tragic tot' Tyra Henry noted that she was in council care. The third day of the case was reported in a brief item on p. 5. After the verdict and sentence the *Daily Express* gave the case the kind of treatment reserved for what are defined as important issues: the whole of pp. 1, 2 and 3 and the entire editorial. A picture of Andrew Neil occupies almost half of the front page under the white-on-black headline 'The monster', with the secondary headlines '"Cannibal Kid" gets life for murder of little Tyra' and 'Did he blind his other child?' (*Daily Express* 26 July 1985). Pages 2 and 3 have two main stories and seven subsidiary items, with pictures of Tyra Henry, Tyrone Henry, Claudette Henry, and the judge in the case. One of the main items is an interview with a 'top detective' by an *Express* crime reporter. The thrust is that, while the police were aware of the dangers to the child, they were thwarted by social workers' and neighbours' fear of the accused. Three other items, 'Now social workers face rap', 'Probe reveals basic blunders' and 'What the judge was not told', reinforce the message that the child's death was preventable. The narrative is framed entirely as the cumulative failure of individuals.

Despite the highly racialized treatment of the case, both in pictures and text, the divisions within the local social services about ethnicity and child protection are not introduced. Instead, the internal reports which focused on individual workers are treated as definitive. (The editorial refs to a 'team of investigators'.) Conversely, the judge's conclusion that social workers should not be blamed is cancelled by a 'senior policeman' saying that the judge 'did not know the full story' (*Daily Express* 26 July 1985) and describing the judge as having 'earned a reputation for leniency, showing mercy to violent offenders'. Mercy is clearly not a virtue in the eyes of the *Daily Express*. Another short item on the page criticizes social services for not helping to pay off Tyra Henry's grandmother's (in whose care she was) electricity bill. Mid-market tabloids are usually more anxious to promote family independence than state support.

The entire 'Express Opinion' is devoted to the case. Its condemnation of social work is comprehensive, ranging from allegedly preventable deaths to the lack of qualifications of residential care workers. Social workers show 'incompetence' and 'bumbling amateurism', are 'fobbed off or fooled'. Towards the end of the piece, the magisterial stance is demonstrated by the balancing statement 'Of course many social workers are qualified. Of course many are wise, compassionate and experienced. And very overworked.' Nevertheless: 'the record suggests many are not. We have a horde of badly qualified or unqualified amateurs, many of whom seem to have gravitated towards social work for want of anything else to do.'

The *Daily Express* reported the NALGO/BASW protests over several days. The report on 27 July was bylined 'Crime Reporter' and on 31 July a large item on p. 10 described a row about the interview with the police officer that had been given major play on 26 July.

On 27 July a dramatic feature appeared: 'Are black power politics costing the lives of children?' The article, about the 'sinister power struggle that has been taking place in Lambeth', 'one of those London boroughs renowned for its "loony left" activities', is described as a 'special report'. While not an explicit 'opinion piece', neither does it fit the canons of 'hard news' because, in what is clearly set out as a conflict, only one side is given space. Although the social services staff were 'bungling bureaucrats' the previous day, professional sources on disagreements with councillors are treated as definitive. There is no balancing account. The report is organized around Janet Boateng (pictured with her small child) as part of an 'activist couple in the front line' with a history of radicalism.

Coverage in the *Daily Mail* was prominent but routine compared with the resources invested by the *Daily Express*. The material is either not bylined or headed 'Daily Mail Reporter', suggesting that the case had not been assigned to a single member of staff. The first day of the trial took up most of p. 5, including three pictures. Two were of Tyra Henry, one when she was healthy, another when in intensive care, and one of Andrew Neil. Days two and three appeared on pp. 14 and 17 respectively. That Tyra was the subject of a care order is mentioned on day three, but is secondary to allegations of perjury.

With the verdict and sentence, the case is suddenly given much greater prominence, becoming the p. 1 lead: 'BABY TYRA: WHAT JUDGE DIDN'T KNOW' in very large (2.5 cm) type. The story is continued on p. 9 where two main items with three pictures fill the page: 'Baby Tyra's brother was blinded in attack'; 'Face of beast who bit his daughter 57 times and murdered her'; 'Social workers' mistakes . . . and clashes' (*Daily Mail* 26 July 1985). The picture of Andrew Neil is in 'mug-shot' style, unlike the more informal view used by the other papers. The main report is a routine round-up of the court proceedings, above a continuation of the p. 1 story, which sketches some of the background. The internal reports are summarized with an indication of the complexity of the issues. Several points of view are mentioned, although more space is given to BASW and the Conservative opposition than to the thinking behind the 'Good Practice Guide' on work with black families.

The same issue gives its first leader to 'Could Baby Tyra have been saved?', with the relatively low-key conclusion that the case merits a 'full and open' public inquiry, 'including not only the council's servants, but its politicians too' (*Daily Mail* 26 July 1985). The following day the paper reported 'Strike as council acts on Tyra' below 'New rules to protect tragic children', on p. 2. The 'rules' are those announced by the junior health minister and are covered without comment by a *Mail* 'political reporter'. The 'Strike' report gets standard 'balanced' coverage as a hard news item. Both are commented upon in another first leader, which opens 'Had the social workers responsible for baby Tyra Henry been more conscientious, she might have been alive today' (*Daily Mail* 27 July 1985). The line taken is that the central government-imposed practice guidelines will ensure that social workers put the interests of children first, regardless of race and 'Left-wing London politicians interfering'.

In the *Daily Mirror* the first day of the Tyra Henry case was given dramatic treatment on p. 5 under the large headline 'A FATHER "BIT BABY 57 TIMES"'. The bylined report includes two pictures: a small shot of Andrew Neil and a much large photo of Tyra Henry in hospital. The *Mirror* news treatment on day two continues in a very similar format: dramatic but neutral in tone. Day three of the trial is not covered. On 26 July the verdict is again the main story on p. 5: 'THE BRUTE GETS LIFE'; 'TRAGIC LIFE OF TYRA'S BLINDED BROTHER'; 'Social workers could face sack'. The word 'brute' is in 6 cm type; there are small pictures of Tyra, Claudette Henry, and Andrew Neil. In the text the details of the court case are outlined, and the Lambeth internal reports described, although with no political background. Allegations of blame against named workers are reproduced, but countered by a NALGO reply. The 'tragic life' is very much in the 'human interest' category, and its second paragraph opens 'A social worker who is helping to ease what is left of the boy's life said. . .'. There was no editorial comment. The NALGO strike was reported on 29 July, together with the announcement of central government guidelines, in a prominent hard news item on p. 2.

In the *Mirror* coverage the 'search for blame' is not an organizing concept; the focus is rather on the human tragedy, with some details of the local professional context. Attributing guilt and psychopathology is, however, a dominant theme of the *Sun*'s presentation. On the opening day of the trial, the picture of Tyra Henry in hospital dominates p. 1 under the strapline 'Horror death of tiny Tyra'. The main headline is 'DAD BIT HIS BABY 57 TIMES!' Inside, the bylined report fills p. 7, headed 'BABY HORROR DAD WENT HOME TO A PARTY' (*Sun* 23 July 1985). There are pictures of Tyra, of Andrew Neil and of his sister Denise shielding Claudette Henry from photographers. On day two the case is the lead on p. 5: 'TRAGIC TYRA WAS "IN CARE"'.

On day three the case was relegated to p. 23, but the conclusion of the trial was given tabloid splash treatment: most of p. 1, a pp. 2–3 spread and leader. A strapline on p. 1, beside a picture of Tyra, reads 'BLUNDERS THAT LED TO BABY'S MURDER' above 'ANIMAL GETS LIFE';'Tyra's dad had already blinded her brother' (*Sun* 26 July 1985). A large mug-shot picture of Andrew Neil, in what is clearly a prison shirt, is captioned 'friends called him The Animal' and the text begins 'Monster Andrew Neil was jailed for life yesterday'. Inside, the theme of individual responsibility is relentlessly pressed home. The double page spread has a white-on-black banner heading 'OUR DEADLY BLUNDERS', below which is 'Social worker in tragic Tyra case quits job'. There are pictures of Tyra on life-support, of the misleading note left with her at hospital, of Denise Neil with Claudette Henry, and of one of the social workers who 'may face disciplinary action'. The main text starts 'Social services chief Stephen Bubb admitted last night that his council blundered badly', rather obscuring that he was vice-chair of the committee. Most of the article repeats those parts of the internal report that were directed at the specific actions of named individuals. There is little indication of the complex practice, political and even racial dimensions. Janet Boateng (see other newspaper coverage) is not mentioned. It concludes with the 'rocket' from 'Lambeth's opposition Tory leader . . . She claimed they lacked one basic skill – common sense'. At the side of the page is a story headed 'Helpless victims of cruel fathers', a rehash of brief details of Jasmine Beckford and Maria Colwell, who were 'tortured and killed by *step*fathers' (my emphasis) for which 'social workers have been blamed before'. Andrew Neil was Tyra Henry's natural father.

In the same edition the *Sun* devotes its whole editorial to the case.

In care? There can rarely have been such a grotesque abuse of the English language . . . Her father Andrew Neil is starting a life sentence that is totally inadequate for his bestial wickedness. But Neil is by no means the only guilty party in this tragedy.

(*Sun* 26 July 1985)

After the standard acknowledgement that social work is 'demanding and difficult', Tyra Henry's death is attributed to the 'catalogue of blunders', the 'mistakes of two women officers', who turned being '"at risk" . . . into a death sentence'. The closing paragraphs read: 'Just when are the authorities going to devise a system for protecting vulnerable children that really works? Just when are they going to ensure that they employ only social workers who know what they are doing and are actually concerned?' Here several potential difficulties are smoothed away: the problem becomes containable; it is rendered into a bureaucratic rather than a social issue; systems are only the aggregate of individuals – if the individuals are competent, then such deaths will be prevented.

On 27 July, 'TYRA STRIKE FURY' ran from a box on p. 1 to another on p. 2, in which the dispute, the trial, and 'Ministers conducting an urgent review on how to slash red tape' are reported.

The inquiry chaired by Stephen Sedley QC reported in December 1987 (Henry 1987). The *Guardian* described its findings in detail in three articles on p. 2 (19 December 1987): 'Tyra "doomed to die before she was born"'; 'Earlier reports failed to solve issue of blame'; 'Social workers castigated for "misjudgements"', linked by the symbolic picture of Tyra Henry on life-support. The reports, together with a second leader, distribute responsibility widely: poor practice; poor supervision; the need for law reform to shift the focus from parent to child. The leader is very critical of NALGO's role in the events, pointing out that social work, although often unfairly castigated, is not above criticism, and that the Sedley report had defended the 'legitimacy, as well as the legal fact, of elected councillors' involvement in the social work process'.

In contrast, the *Daily Telegraph* covered the report as a

straightforward news item, leading p. 2 (18 December). The story opens 'Misjudgements and incompetence by social workers are blamed', and then moves on to a brief summary of the report and some of the background. The concluding section is a balancing response from NALGO, characterizing the report as 'scapegoating yet another social worker' when the problem is resources.

The *Daily Express* account of the inquiry appeared as a bylined report on p. 7, illustrated with part of the 'hospital picture'. Despite the emotive tone of the opening, which speaks of 'bitter recriminations' and 'tragic conclusions' (*Daily Express* 19 December 1987), the rest of the text is in hard news style with a variety of perspectives reported.

The treatment of the report in both the *Daily Mail* and the *Daily Mirror* on 18 December 1987 is unusual. Both place the item on p. 5 with some prominence, including a small picture of Tyra Henry when healthy. In their different styles they summarize the report as identifying a range of causes including individual poor practice, incorrect priorities and inadequate liaison between housing and social services. Phrases like 'is expected' strongly suggest that the basis of the stories is a press release. On 19 December there are further reports, presumably based on a sight of the actual document. The *Daily Mail*'s account (in a box on p. 9) is headed 'The woman who failed tragic Tyra', below a strapline 'CHILD ABUSE: SOCIAL WORKER ACCUSED AS LIST OF SHAME GROWS'. Half the story focuses on the blame attached to a named worker, the rest to brief background details and a comment from NALGO. In similar fashion, perhaps in a parallel search for 'closure', the *Daily Mirror* ran a second story on 19 December (in a box on p. 2 with the same picture) highlighting the failures of practice and the implied contradiction that no disciplinary action was to be taken.

The *Sun* did not cover the report of the inquiry.

THE CHARLENE SALT CASE

In October 1985 David Salt was tried at Manchester Crown Court for the manslaughter and ill-treatment of his daughter Charlene Salt, aged 3 months. The trial lasted nine days; at its conclusion David Salt, who had pleaded not guilty, was found guilty on both charges and sentenced to six years' imprisonment. Gail Salt, Charlene's mother, was also tried and convicted of neglect. She was sentenced to three years' probation. Both David and Gail Salt are white.

The *Guardian* covered the case throughout, although not every day. The first day's proceedings were the first lead on p. 2, with considerable detail, but no byline, suggesting that the material had come from an agency or perhaps the *Manchester Evening News*, which is part of the same organization. The story opened: 'A three and a half month old baby girl who slept in a closed drawer at night if she cried died despite the efforts of eight experts who knew she was at risk' (*Guardian* 22 October 1985). Later paragraphs focused on the policy and professional dimensions of the case, reproducing the prosecuting counsel's assertion that the welfare agencies had been thwarted by '"a combination of sheer misfortune and the cunning of David Salt, who set out to deceive them"'. The verdict and sentence were reported by the *Guardian* at the top of p. 5 with two items (neither with byline) grouped with four pictures, of Charlene Salt, David Salt, the Director of Oldham Social Services and (in a much bigger shot) Gail Salt beside the infamous chest of drawers. As much space was given to 'Council reviews "at risk" system' as to a summary of the case (*Guardian* 1 November 1985). There was no editorial comment.

Coverage in the *Daily Telegraph* was confined to the first day of the trial and its final outcome. The account of the first day was given moderate prominence on p. 3, again without a byline. It opens 'A 3-month-old baby girl who died after being roughly shaken by her father had been on a social services "at risk" register' and continued with a broad summary both of the work of the agencies involved and the dramatically squalid domestic circumstances (*Daily Telegraph* 22 October 1985). The report of the end of the trial appeared as a bylined article leading p. 2: 'Baby in drawer killer jailed for six years'. After summarizing the trial, the conclusion of a departmental review, that staff and procedures had not been at fault, is reported. The family's social worker, appearing at a press conference, is quoted: '"Professionally I feel I did everything possible. As a woman and a mother I feel absolutely grief-stricken and devastated"' (*Daily Telegraph* 1 November 1985). There was no leader comment.

The first day of the trial was reported on as the main story on p. 10 of the *Daily Express*, bylined 'Express Reporter', and beginning, 'The cunning of brutal father David Salt foiled attempts by a team of social workers and doctors to see his baby daughter, a court heard yesterday' (*Daily Express* 22 October 1985). The main emphasis of the rest of the story is the extent of the professional support offered. There were no further reports until the conclusion of the case when the *Express* gave over most of p. 5 to 'Baby-in-drawer killer jailed for six years', below the strapline 'Wife walks free from death court and vows to divorce "monster"' (1 November 1985). The coverage includes two news items, small pictures of David Salt and Gail Salt, and a much larger photograph of Charlene in her cot. The bylined news report is a brief summary of the circumstances and the sentence. Part of the concluding section reads

> More than a dozen child care experts were involved in her case after she was found to be at risk at the age of two weeks. But their efforts were thwarted by a combination of misfortune and the deception of Salt.

> (*Daily Express*, 1 November 1985)

Yet the other piece of text, not bylined and presumably based on the social services press conference, is headlined 'Care boss admits: We made mistake'. This is based on the director's expression of regret that Charlene was not taken into care, rather than placed under supervision. Although his declaration that all concerned had acted properly is reported, the whole inflection is the culpability of individuals. 'Experts' decided against the 'safe custody' of a care order; the social worker's office was 'just three doors away from the baby's home'.

The *Sun* reported the first day of the case on p. 7 in a bylined account, quoting prosecuting counsel and describing social workers as having 'won a court order for her safety' (*Sun* 22 October 1985). Two further reports appeared during the proceedings, both focused on the family's home and the personality of David Salt: '"I strangled cat" says Dad' (*Sun* 29 October 1985). The verdict and sentence got dramatic but not extended treatment, appearing on pp. 1 and 2. 'Drawer of death', in 4.5 cm white-on-black type, was followed by 'Fury as baby killer gets only 6 years'. The front page story included a large picture of Gail Salt beside the chest of drawers and a smaller picture of Charlene; the p. 2 continuation is organized around the theme of David Salt's deviance and culpability: he is 'Long-haired', 'domineering', cruel to animals, violent and 'sly'. A picture of him with Charlene is captioned 'Bath-time . . . Salt holds Charlene by the neck' (*Sun* 1 November 1985). The Director of Oldham Social Services is quoted as saying '"We all feel now that we failed Charlene" But he added . . . "We have to take risks in sending children home, otherwise we would have thousands in care." '

The *Daily Mirror*'s reports of the case were framed within the same news values as those of the *Sun*, but given much greater 'play' throughout. Day one of the case was give splash coverage. The headline 'SHUT IN A DRAWER FOR CRYING' (*Daily Mirror* 22 October 1985) together with a big picture of Charlene Salt, the 'Tiny victim of "torture"', and a small picture of David Salt occupied most of the front page. The bylined report continued on p. 7, as 'AGONY OF BABY CHARLENE' in 3 cm type and illustrated with small pictures of the baby and Gail Salt. Again the theme is that David Salt was 'so cunning' as to able to 'fool' an 'experienced team'. Four days of proceedings were reported, emphasizing the filthy home conditions and the accused's violent behaviour. On 30 October Gail Salt's emotional accusation of her husband was the main story on p. 5 with white-on-black headline: '"YOU MURDERER!"'

Almost four pages were given over to the outcome of the case: most of p. 1, a continuation and editorial on p. 2, and a double page spread on pp. 4 and 5. The front page is dominated by a picture of David Salt knitting a charity blanket, in a box labelled 'MIRROR EXCLUSIVE' with the headline 'HANDS THAT KILLED BABY CHARLENE' below the strapline 'Evil father gets six years'. Most of the news report focuses on the reaction of relatives, the MP for a neighbouring constituency and a paediatrician calling for a longer sentence on 'the brute'. Also on p. 2, the 'Mirror comment' declares 'Again and again we have demanded measures to give children the greater protection which is their right . . . The punishment should fit the crime. Six years (or possibly less) for David Salt does no such thing' (*Daily Mirror* 1 November 1985).

On pp. 4 and 5, there are two motifs: human interest and the search for blame. Charlene Salt is pictured in her cot and her '105 days of pain and torment' set out in a miserable chronology. The pages are dominated by the headline 'ALL THESE PEOPLE CARED BUT BABY CHARLENE STILL DIED IN MISERY'. Bisecting the headline is a row of women's faces: the health visitor, three social workers and four neighbours who 'cared'. At the foot of the page is another item about the 'callous and uncaring . . . monster', whose 'jealousy bordered on madness' and who 'made frequent demands for kinky sex'. David Salt is constructed as not only abnormal, but obviously so. The effect of this is to neutralize his alleged slyness and cunning, used in other accounts to explain the failure of official systems. Indeed the *Daily Mirror* version, which is clearly the outcome of some investigative effort as three people are bylined, makes almost no reference at all to the complex agency background, involving doctors, hospitals, the probation service, etc. The 'local bobby' is mentioned in the text, but he is not pictured. The scenario is transformed into a failure of professional women to listen to the common sense of the women neighbours – who themselves should have been more decisive – in this everyday family melodrama.

It was obvious from the start that evil David Salt and his educationally subnormal wife Gail were hopelessly inadequate to bring up a new baby . . . Salt's violent nature was an open secret among concerned neighbours [who] watched helplessly as they saw a procession of social workers knock on the Salts' door but get no answer even though the couple were at home.

(*Daily Mirror* 1 November 1985)

The *Daily Mirror* as a mildly Labour paper thus manages to avoid a simple attack on the welfare state while inviting readers to agree that ordinary folk like themselves know wrongdoing when they see it.

The trial was, of course, major news locally. The *Evening Chronicle* of Oldham reported the case on p. 1 every day, often continuing the coverage on an inside page. During the trial the involvement of welfare professionals was not a major theme; much more space was given to the rehearsal of events, the character and behaviour of David Salt, Gail Salt's accusations against him, and his allegation that the police had ill-treated him. The articles were in plain descriptive format, plainly set out.

On 31 October the verdict and sentence took most of p. 1 of the *Evening Chronicle*: 'SALT IS JAILED FOR 6 YEARS', beside a picture of Charlene Salt. On p. 3 there is an elaborate 'special report' by three reporters which, headed 'We can't play God', sets an internally consistent interpretative framework for allocating blame. There are four articles and an editorial 'comment'. Two of the articles explore the guilt feelings of neighbours and the behaviour of David Salt. Although Salt is described as a 'brutal bully' with a reputation for violent lawless behaviour, he is not depicted as an asocial grotesque. The more bizarre details of the Salts' domestic life are given little space, compared with the national press accounts. In a further short but prominent piece a local paediatrician expresses the rather ambivalent view that although 'he cannot apportion blame' child deaths are preventable because "We are making fundamental errors in our approach [by] treating the symptoms, not the causes".' He does not say what the causes are.

Most of the space in the main story is given to the senior assistant director of social services, but her assertion that blame must ultimately rest with the parents is set within a text where she 'admits' and the opening paragraph announces, 'Baby Charlene would probably still be alive today if high-ranking welfare staff in Oldham had not decided that she ought to stay at home with her parents.' All these narratives fit with the leader, which heads the page. While acknowledging that 'There can be no excusing' the behaviour of the Salts, it asserts that 'warning signs were obvious' but not acted upon. But having made the strong statement that 'Charlene could have been rescued from her most horrible fate by the very system that in the end turned its back on her' the writer then retreats

and widens the net of fault to 'neighbours and relatives' as well as professionals, concluding that such events can be prevented 'if the rest of us, the
amateurs, heed the terrified cry in the night and watch our neighbours for
the danger signs'.

The same ambivalence about locating cause in individuals or
collectivities, whether the community or official agencies, also emerges
in a follow-up the next day 'CHARLENE: THE AFTERMATH'
(*Evening Chronicle* 1 November 1985). Reporting the family social
workers's appearance at the press conference, the page is headed 'I FEEL
DEVASTATED; Salt care worker did "everything possible"'. A further
report makes clear that both the social services department and the
committee had investigated and were satisfied with their findings.
Nevertheless the social worker, who is reported as feeling she had acted
properly, is linguistically transformed into being on the defensive. She
'admits', 'confesses', 'denies'. Despite the obvious attempt by the local
authority to make a positive and coherent response to the case, and the
close involvement of other social services and health care workers, the
family's social worker has become the centre of attention. In the search
for a simplifying framework and satisfactory closure, she provides an
obvious focus.

THE REUBEN CARTHY CASE

In December 1985, Maureen Ricketts was tried at Nottingham Crown
Court for the manslaughter of her son Reuben Junior Carthy, aged 2 years,
and for actual bodily harm and his wilful ill-treatment. She pleaded not
guilty to all charges. The boy's father, Reuben Carthy, was also on trial
for actual bodily harm and wilful ill-treatment, to which he pleaded
guilty. At the conclusion of the four-day hearing, Maureen Ricketts was
sentenced to four years' imprisonment for manslaughter and Reuben
Carthy to eighteen months' imprisonment. Both Maureen Ricketts and
Reuben Carthy are African-Caribbean.

The only national coverage of the Carthy case was of the verdict and
sentence. *The Times* had a short descriptive item on p. 3 mentioning that,
ten days before her son died, Maureen Ricketts had told her GP that she
was hitting him.

The *Daily Express* reported the trial in a brief (10 cm) factual item at
the foot of p. 2.

Maureen Ricketts's statements that she had tried to get help were
prominent in the *Daily Mirror*'s brief account, 'Four years for killer
mother', at the foot of p. 7: 'A young mother who killed her two-year-old

son after pleading for help from social workers was jailed for four years yesterday. Maureen Ricketts, 21, told social services she was hitting the boy and was worried that she might hurt him' (*Daily Mirror* 19 December 1985). The *Sun* also reported the outcome of the case on p. 7: 'Mother punched boy to death'; 'Evil Mum Maureen was jailed for four years yesterday' (*Sun* 19 December 1985). The bylined account describes the boy's injuries, the comments of the judge and the demeanour of the accused, but does not draw attention to the involvement of doctors and social workers.

The *Guardian* did not report the case at all.

None of the papers sampled made any editorial comment.

THE STEPHANIE FOX CASE

In March 1990, Stephen Fox was tried at the Old Bailey for the murder of his daughter Stephanie, aged 3 years. At the conclusion of the case, which lasted five days, Stephen Fox, who had pleaded not guilty, was convicted of murder and sentenced to life imprisonment. Stephen Fox is white.

Only *The Independent*, of the papers sampled, reported the trial when it was in progress, once, in a brief descriptive account on p. 3.

The *Daily Telegraph* reported the verdict and sentence in three one-sentence paragraphs on p. 3. The second paragraph reads 'Stephen Fox ... denied murdering Stephanie, who was on Wandsworth social services department's "at risk" register' (*Daily Telegraph* 31 March 1990). *The Independent* also included this feature of the case in the second paragraph of its account. Although a longer item than the *Telegraph*'s and placed on p. 2, the item has no byline and no illustrations.

The *Sun*, under the headline 'Dad who shook tot to death gets life' (*Sun* 31 March 1990) gave the case 8 cm of text on p. 4. That the child was in care is not mentioned; the last paragraph reads 'Last night the local council child care committee promised a full enquiry.'

The *Daily Mirror* did not report the case.

Only the *Daily Mail* gave the case prominent coverage. Leading p. 9, and illustrated by a small picture of Stephanie Fox, the headline 'Murdered girl was in danger all her life' (*Daily Mail* 31 March 1990) clearly signals the interpretative framework. Although the story is bylined as from a named 'Chief Reporter', there is nothing in the text that could not have been derived from agency reports of the trial. The style falls somewhere between hard news and 'colour':

Little Stephanie Fox never had a chance . . . when she was three she died at the hands of the drunken father she so feared . . . It happened despite the fact that she spent most of her life on a council's 'at risk' register, despite constant signs of physical and personal abuse also noted by social workers and despite calls for increased vigilance after a series of child abuse scandals . . . Last night Wandsworth social services launched an urgent enquiry into why she was not taken into protective custody.

(*Daily Mail* 31 March 1990)

The account goes on to characterize Stephen Fox as an obvious deviant and to catalogue the social services' actions in the case.

The internal inquiry was indeed 'urgent'; it reported in June 1990 (Fox 1990). The national press response was interestingly asymmetrical from that devoted to the original trial. The *Daily Telegraph* provided a detailed account of the inquiry report, leading p. 3 and including two pictures, of Stephanie Fox and of Stephen Fox. The headline and opening paragraph reads 'Social workers failed to save battered girl':

Social workers failed to save the life of a three-year-old girl by taking her into care even though it was known that she had been injured on 30 separate occasions, an independent report into the death last August of Stephanie Fox announced yesterday.

(*Daily Telegraph* 21 June 1990)

Yet the second paragraph continues 'The report also said that a shortage of Wandsworth Council staff may have contributed to her death' and the rest of the account centres on the department's resource problems, resulting vacant posts, slowness to react, and failures of communication. Half-way down the first column of the three-column report it is observed that the borough is a 'Tory flagship with the lowest poll tax in England'.

The Independent's version is rolled up into a p. 3 section on the consequences of the poll tax and concludes with a comment from Labour's social services spokesman. The *Sun* takes the same line, in its p. 11 lead: 'POLL TAX CASH CUTS "LED TO TODDLER'S DEATH"; Steph, 3, missed out on care' (*Sun* 21 June 1990). Beside a small picture of the child, the hard news item opens

Cash cuts under a Tory council poll tax budget helped lead to the death of three-year-old Stephanie Fox, an inquiry revealed yesterday . . . Social workers knew she was at risk and wanted her safely looked after at a day centre. But the London borough where Stephanie lived reduced its care facilities after setting a poll tax of £148, the lowest in England.

(*Sun* 21 June 1990)

The report concludes with a denial that further cuts are planned. Clearly the news treatment of an issue cannot always be simply 'read off' from the politics of the newspaper concerned.

The *Daily Mirror*'s report contained the same message, but condensed into three paragraphs at the foot of p. 2: 'Cash cuts "linked" to tot's death' (*Daily Mirror* 21 June 1990).

The *Daily Mail* did not report the inquiry's findings.

THE TRACY WILKINSON CASE

In October 1990 Anita Wilkinson and Benjamin Gaskin were tried at Sheffield Crown Court after the death of Tracy Wilkinson at the age of 15 months. Anita Wilkinson pleaded guilty to manslaughter by neglect and was jailed for five years. Benjamin Gaskin, Anita Wilkinson's partner, denied murder. He was found guilty and sentenced to life imprisonment. Both Anita Wilkinson and Benjamin Gaskin are white.

Of the national papers sampled, the *Daily Mirror*, the *Daily Telegraph* and the *Sun* did not cover the case. (The *Sun* had other preoccupations on the day after the verdict and sentence: pp. 1, 2 and 3 were given over to 'UP YOURS DELORS' and more along the same lines.) *The Independent* mentioned the trial outcome in a one-paragraph item in a p. 2 news round-up.

The *Guardian* report, under the headline 'Life for man who beat up and killed toddler' as one of the main items on p. 3 (*Guardian* 1 November 1990), highlights the comments of the judge about the respective culpability of the two accused and the part played by the NSPCC, who had been involved with the family. It concludes with a statement from the NSPCC that two officers had been '"spoken to"' and that policies had been reviewed.

Only the *Daily Mail* gave the case prominent treatment, with an illustrated report as the lead on p. 5. There are three pictures, two small mug-shot-style views of the accused, and a much larger picture of the child's cot, captioned 'TRAGIC TRACY'S TORTURE ROOM'. Benjamin Gaskin is described as a 'sadistic sex offender' but his personality and behaviour, the sordid domestic conditions, and the limited intelligence of Anita Wilkinson (all of which parallel the Charlene Salt case) are not highlighted. The main theme is identified in the headline:

'NSPCC "lost" toddler locked in attic to die' (*Daily Mail* 1 November 1990). The NSPCC, who 'admitted last night that it had lost contact for 20 days with a tragic toddler whose welfare it was monitoring', are described as being 'fobbed off' by the child's mother. There is, though, almost no development of the NSPCC's blameworthiness and it is left to their spokesman to close the matter:

> The main lesson for us is that we have to be more persistent and insistent on satisfying ourselves about a child's welfare. But you cannot live with these families 24 hours a day, and we rely a great deal on trust and co-operation.
>
> (*Daily Mail* 1 November 1990)

The *Daily Mail* did not make any leader comment on the case.

The Tracy Wilkinson case had a number of features reminiscent of previous high-profile instances. Social work practice and procedures had admittedly fallen short. According to *Community Care* (8 November 1990), the episode had been the subject of a social services department internal inquiry which had been critical of the NSPCC, to the extent of 'considering monitoring NSPCC casework'. Of the two workers highlighted in press accounts, one was a student, which one might have expected neatly to combine the mid-market tabloid's recurrent motifs of bungling management and inadequately equipped front-line staff. Yet national press interest ranged from relatively low-key to nil.

THE SUDIO ROUSE CASE

In a trial at the Old Bailey lasting throughout October 1991, Robert Rouse and Lindsay Morris were accused of the murder of their daughter Sudio Rouse, aged 6 weeks, and of cruelty to their other daughter, 'Baby Y', then aged 2 years. Lindsay Morris was acquitted of murder on the direction of the judge and then pleaded guilty to the other charges. She was remanded for reports. Robert Rouse admitted one of the charges relating to Baby Y, but pleaded not guilty to the other offences. At the conclusion of the case, he was acquitted of one of the charges relating to Baby Y but convicted of another charge of cruelty to her, of cruelty to Sudio Rouse, and of the murder of Sudio Rouse. He was sentenced to life imprisonment. (Both defendants subsequently lodged an appeal.) Robert Rouse and Lindsay Morris are white.

The Times presented the first day of the trial dramatically. The case appears in a box at the top of p. 3, with pictures, strapline, and byline, headed 'Pair "murdered baby by banging her head on bedroom wall"'

(*The Times* 3 October 1991) (although, as described above, only Robert Rouse was convicted of murder and he subsequently appealed.) There are large photographs of the accused and a smaller shot of a doctor called by the prosecution although, oddly, the text does not quote the substance of her evidence. Despite the initial play, there was no further coverage of the case in *The Times*.

The Independent gave the opening of the case considerable prominence as the lead story on p. 3, with two pictures. Further reports followed on days two and three – short accounts, both on p. 7. The outcome formed the lead on p. 5: 'Father gets life for murder of baby daughter' (*The Independent* 31 October 1991). The bylined article is illustrated with two small pictures of the accused and is presented in straight factual style. Equal space is given to an account of the circumstances leading to the baby's death, and to the background issue that both children had been on the 'at risk' register of the London Borough of Croydon. The director is quoted as saying that the baby's death was '"deeply regrettable"' but he 'insisted that social workers followed proper procedures to protect her'. There was no leader comment.

Nothing appeared in the *Daily Mail* until the end of the trial, when it was reported on p. 5 that 'Cruel father gets life for killing baby Sudio', below the strapline 'SISTERS BATTERED AND BITTEN IN CATALOGUE OF TORTURE'. A further inset sub-headline reads 'We weren't to blame says social work chief' (*Daily Mail* 31 October 1991). Both of the accused and Sudio Rouse are pictured. The story opens with the aspect of the circumstances brought out in much of the coverage:

> A wicked father began a life sentence last night for murdering his baby by smashing her against a wall. Robert Rouse picked up six-week-old Sudio by the ankle and swung her with such force that her skull was fractured and the wall was dented.
>
> (*Daily Mail* 31 October 1991)

After a brief account of the legal aspects of the case, the grim details of the injuries to Sudio and Baby Y are described. The latter half of the article is a chronology of events from Baby Y's being put under a care order and placed with foster parents in 1989, after contact between the local hospital, the police and social services.

> The decision to return [Baby Y] was made after the couple had shown interest in her welfare and visited her regularly. They even attended classes to improve their skills as parents. Social services *took the*

precaution of putting the child on the 'At Risk' register, which should have ensured that she was watched closely.

(Daily Mail 31 October 1991; my emphasis)

The story ends with the director's statement that 'proper procedures' had been followed. The *Daily Mail* made no editorial comment on the case.

In the *Daily Mirror*, the first day of the case was the bylined main story on p. 17 with the dramatic white-on-black headline 'BABY BASHED SO HARD SHE DENTED THE WALL' and pictures of both the accused (*Daily Mirror* 3 October 1991). Nothing more appeared until 24 October, when there was a short report of the acquittal of Lindsay Morris on the murder charge, again on p. 17. On 31 October the outcome of the case filled most of p. 17: 'LET MY TRAGIC LITTLE SUDIO BE LAID TO REST NOW'. This, a strapline and a sub-headline focused on a dispute between the parents' families about paying for the baby's funeral. The dramatic presentation includes a large picture of Robert Rouse, and smaller pictures of Sudio Rouse, 'Cruel mum: Morris' and 'Centre of the storm: The mortuary at Croydon'. Apart from the opening 'angle' on the family dispute, there is a broadly factual account of the circumstances of the case and the actions of official agencies. Robert Rouse and Lindsay Morris are described as 'tormentors' and he as a 'brute', but some of the more ghastly aspects of the case are offset by details which underline her limited abilities and his ineffectual attempts to do the right thing. Robert Rouse is not transformed by the news coverage into a monster.

The agency background is also introduced: 'doctors and social workers clashed over their failings ... DOCTORS said they were too overworked to take proper action. SOCIAL WORKERS said the doctors had been duped by the baby's parents.' In the concluding sections 'doctors hit out at Health Service shortages which meant that battered babies were seen by different experts who did not have time to co-ordinate reports' and the statement by the director of social services was quoted.

On day one of the trial, the *Sun* gave most of p. 13 to the case: '"PARENTS KILLED BABY BY KNOCKING A DENT IN A WALL WITH ITS HEAD"; It was plugged with Polyfilla, murder jury told' (*Sun* 3 October 1991). Both the accused are pictured, and the details put before the court reported in 60 column cm of text – very extensive by *Sun* standards. As the case continued, the only further item was on the acquittal of Lindsay Morris on the murder charge. The *Sun* (31 October 1991) confined its report of the outcome of the Sudio Rouse case to 'Tot killer is jailed for life' – five descriptive paragraphs on p. 15.

INTERPRETING THE NEWS TREATMENT

Transforming events into news is often termed 'manufacture' or 'production'. The trouble with these partly metaphorical terms is that they are highly mechanistic: macho imagery which fits the professional ideology of newsgatherers and academic theorists alike. A better metaphor for media organizations is that they are restaurants: highly sensitive to the market, with a known cuisine and style imprint. But recipes never come out the same way twice, and this year's passion may be relegated as boring next.

Thus, when someone is put on trial for the death of a child who was in the care of social services, the probability of the case figuring prominently in the national press increases with the number of certain specific 'ingredients' present (which is another way of understanding Galtung and Ruge's (1965) image of 'amplitude' described in Chapter 1). But their availability does not completely determine the detail of the news treatment – or even that the case will be reported.

National newspapers are (or try to be) highly responsive to their sector of the market. Broadsheet readers are defined as holding positions of minor or major responsibility in key social institutions: industry; commerce; health, welfare, education and other public services; the polity. The mass tabloids address those whose autonomy is restricted to their leisure and domestic life. Mid-market, one might speculate, are those who hold positions of some responsibility but little power – and often resent it. As we have seen from the press coverage, the case of a dead child for whom social services had responsibility is likely to have aspects which could fit the imperatives of any or all newspapers – and yet apparently similar scenarios attract very different treatment.

So what are the ingredients which make it more likely that such an instance will be reported, by which papers and within what interpretative framework? I shall argue that the episodes discussed above demonstrate a clear pattern. The most intense national press coverage has been focused on those cases which were constructed as self-evidently major news, because they 'scored' on all the key ingredients: a certain form of proceedings; a specific place; a key time; having an ethnic dimension; and fitting news values in terms of presentation. The fewer of these, the more that dealing with the story appears to depend on the editorial policy (and politics) of specific newspapers.

- *Style*: The style of the coverage relates to the newspaper's editorial policies and market niche. As we have seen from the coverage itself, 'style' embraces both surface features – pictures, headlines, language and length of text – and the causal model embedded in the narrative.

- *Length of proceedings*: Cases of a few days seem to be more amenable to coverage. They can be planned in as 'continuing news' and there will be time for some investigative work, obtaining photographs, accounts from neighbours, etc., without loss of momentum. Even a very dramatic case may get cursory coverage at its conclusion if it is spread over weeks, as was the Sudio Rouse trial. By extension, one must assume that the defendant(s) must plead not guilty to at least some of the charges. A guilty plea eliminates most of the materials of evidence, counsels' submissions, judge's summing up, upon which press coverage is built.

- *Place*: Among the cases that social workers repeat in their litany of 'bad news', London and the south-east of England are heavily over-represented, for a number of intersecting reasons. Covering a story with the paper's own staff (as opposed to using agency materials or stringers) is expensive, and the more so the further from the office. It is also clear from daily consumption (although very hard to verify) that the national newspapers are very London-centric, both in literal physical terms and culturally. Tripe and whippets start in south Bedfordshire; deviancy is assumed to be endemic among the outlaws of the periphery. But, more importantly, London also stands for a wider political context.

- *Historic/political context*: It is also clear that there was a clustering of intensely covered cases in the mid-1980s – Jasmine Beckford, Kimberley Carlile, Tyra Henry. Equally we have seen above cases like Reuben Carthy and Charlene Salt which, during the same period, received little national press interest, let alone attracting vitriolic leading articles. This was the peak not only of the Thatcher administration's triumphalism but also of Labour opposition through local government.

Although municipal socialism was an active force in the regions, only Liverpool and London attracted sustained national media attention. Interest was intense, as in many areas old Labour Party machines were being replaced by alliances linking the new claims of radical class, race and gender politics: a self-evident anathema to the Tory press, but barely congenial to the centre left of the *Daily Mirror* or the *Guardian* either. Rubbishing the 'loony left' was a very high-profile theme among the Tory mass- and mid-market tabloids from the early 1980s on. Tales about the banning of black bin liners and the nursery rhyme 'Baa Baa Black Sheep' were reproduced with little regard for the usual conventions of 'standing

a story up'. The provenance of these and other fictional stories is described in a report by the Media Research Group (1987). (See Chippindale
and Horrie (1990) and Hollingsworth (1985) for further background.)
What better peg than circumstances capable of interpretation as local
authority failure at every level from zealot committee chair, through
bungling senior officials, to front-line layabouts, full of sociological
claptrap entailing underdeveloped notions of individual responsibility?

The Jasmine Beckford, Kimberley Carlile and Tyra Henry cases all
took place in left-wing London boroughs. Conversely (although more
recently) the less-reported Stephanie Fox and Sudio Rouse cases involved
the social services of two Tory London boroughs. In the case of Stephanie
Fox, the subsequent inquiry was, by implication, highly critical of the
spending priorities of Wandsworth, a supposed model of modern Tory
financial rectitude. The papers most hostile to local authority social work
are the mid-market tabloids, as we have seen. The *Daily Mail* dealt with
this problem by not reporting the outcome of the inquiry. Its treatment of
the Sudio Rouse case is also uncharacteristically mild. Not only is there
no hostile leading article, but the assurances of the director that internal
inquiries have resolved any failures of practice or procedure are accepted,
even given prominence, without question. Where are the demands for the
publication of the 'secret' report which, according to the *Observer* (24
November 1991) was both lengthy and critical? The substance of the
Mail's coverage underlines the extent of the work done, rather than
mistakes made.

The Stephanie Fox case also cautions against too mechanistic a
conception of the editorial process. Would one have expected the *Sun* to
reproduce the inquiry's criticisms? Why did it do so? Because 'tragic tot'
was more salient to its readers? Because supporting the Tories did not
extend to the impact of the poll tax on its working-class audience? Or
because the item, compiled from a press release or agency input, slipped
through the editorial net on to p. 11?

In the other cases under scrutiny the local political set-up does not
feature on the national news agenda. There is no clue as to which party
held power in Oldham during the Charlene Salt case, for instance.

• *Racial dimension*: The coverage of the Tyra Henry case was not only
  racialized but racist: there is no other construction that can be put on
  the recurrent use of photographs of the accused and other participants
  in the case, let alone on appellations like the 'animal' (*Sun* 26 July
  1985) or 'the cannibal kid' (*Daily Express* 26 July 1985). White men
  who carry out attacks of such severity are described as human 'evil' or

'wicked brutes', or as crypto- human or even super-human 'monsters', but rarely as sub-human.

(A third-party complaint was made to the Press Council about *The Times*'s coverage of the Tyra Henry case. The complaint was rejected on the grounds that the 'story was a retrospective report on an already widely publicized case. Photographs of the man had already been published widely' (*The Times* 11 December 1985). Indeed they had; the adjudication provides an insight into the reasons for the demise of the Press Council.)

Yet even for the right-wing press the race of the accused is not by itself a determining factor in picking up a case. In December 1985, a few months after the Tyra Henry hysteria, the Reuben Carthy case was, as we have seen, hardly mentioned in the national press. It is impossible to tell from what did appear that both defendants were black. In the high-profile trials race is, in part, a complex surrogate for other items on the press agenda. One is the racial dimension of the demonized 'loony left' discussed above. Another is the search for the deviant, undeserving, dangerous minority at whom the strong state can legitimately direct its control measures. Andrew Neil was made to stand for the twice-alien, both a moral outcast and the racial 'enemy within'. (See, apart from Hall *et al.* (1978) considered in Chapter 1, van Dijk (1991), Gordon and Rosenberg (1989), Hollingsworth (1985) and Searle (1987), on the treatment of immigrants and then black Britons in the press.) The template – 'violent uncontrolled black man, fearful and inept white social worker, chaotic socialist local authority' – had been set up only a few months beforehand, during the Jasmine Beckford case (Wroe 1988). Thus not only politics but news values and routines made it inevitable that the trial would be extensively reported.

The Tyra Henry case involved issues of ethnicity at every level: both the child's parents were African-Caribbean, as were many neighbours. The trial brought into the public domain the intense pre-existing local controversy about the appropriateness of child protection practices, developed by a mainly white profession from work with predominantly white clients, for the circumstances and cultural practices of other ethnic groups. In turn, this had highlighted the permanent tension between elected members and the professional staff of local authorities in a new and dramatic form. Further, questions were being raised about the 'politicization' of local authorities not merely in the sense of party-political divisions over policy, but claims that senior staff were being appointed on the basis of their political sympathies. All these gave the racial aspects of the Tyra Henry case particular salience for the broadsheet press, whatever its political alignment. Thus these contextual issues received almost as much attention in their reports as the trial itself.

In the mass tabloids the context was down-played. Part of the explanation for this must lie in normal framing practices. Issues are refracted in the mass tabloids through specific persons, where possible, to achieve simplicity, drama, and identification. Social and political structures and processes are abstract and intangible, making for dull coverage. Thus, while the *Daily Mirror* made an attempt briefly to indicate that there was a policy background, the *Sun* simply omitted it, despite the (presumably) inviting target of Janet Boateng.

To have introduced the local politics of race would also, crucially, have messed up the appealingly simple narrative structure in both the *Sun* and the *Daily Express* of 'father kills baby because incompetent, wet lefty social workers had no common sense'. The *Sun* wanted to keep the story simple because that is its stock in trade. For the *Daily Express* one must infer a more complex equation. It is Tory, *petit bourgeois* and tends to white nationalism, but if the political and policy disputes had been introduced into the news stories about the Tyra Henry case, then the possibility would have arisen that social workers' 'mistakes' were not due solely to their personal failings combined with the fundamental misguidedness of the social work mission. It would be hard to avoid either diluting the blame attached to the professionals, or accepting that the local black politicians had a point in their attempts to redirect child protection practice. The *Express* dealt with this contradiction, as noted above, by hiving off the local politics into a feature, separated by time and format from the news coverage, in which it took a completely different stance on professional expertise claims.

- *News values*: The *Daily Mail*'s coverage of the Tyra Henry case was relatively low-key and equivocal for the paper that is usually quickest to find and condemn instances of alleged social work failure. It almost got caught in the 'my enemy's enemy is my friend' dilemma sidestepped by the *Express*. But in other instances examined, like the Stephanie Fox and Tracy Wilkinson cases, the *Daily Mail* gave the cases noticeably greater 'play' than other papers. This nicely illustrates that in explaining lower-profile news treatment, the news values of particular papers are an important factor. Of the papers sampled, one might infer that the *Guardian* was attracted to the Tracy Wilkinson case by the questions raised about voluntary sector social work. Why did the *Daily Mail* give it space? One reason is likely to be the paper's general orientation to social work stories, reinforced by the dramatic details of the particular case. They had also acquired a picture; which came first is an interesting question. 'Blame' is clear, but the NSPCC is not condemned wholesale. This is consistent with another aspect of the *Mail*'s agenda. It is not so much that it is suspicious of social work as of *state* social work – part of the expensive socialist-inspired and dominated welfare bureaucracy. Voluntary agencies are different, as we shall see in Chapter 6.

A paper's internal priorities will determine what resources to devote to a story. Once committed, they need to be justified by extensive play. It is noticeable how much more space the *Daily Mirror* gave to the Charlene Salt case than other papers. Being a mass tabloid it does not disdain drama and human interest, but it distinguishes itself from the *Sun* by being pro-Labour, family-orientated, for slightly older 'folks', and by trying to avoid racism (Andrew Neil was merely a 'brute' (*Daily Mirror* 26 July 1985)). The 'exclusive' picture of David Salt knitting (*Daily Mirror* 1 November 1985) was, presumably, one outcome of the resources allocated to the case from day one, signalled by the bylined report.

Certainly anything that is 'exclusive' seems to affect whether a marginal story is covered at all, or pursued after day one. The *Daily Mirror* demonstrated this, too, with its fresh (and very tabloid human interest) angle on the conclusion of the Sudio Rouse case (*Daily Mirror* 31 October 1991). The low priority given to this by other national dailies presumably reflects not only how long the proceedings had lasted, but that the most dramatic symbol, of the dented wall, emerged on day one and was not superseded by anything more simple and powerful. Even broadsheet papers seem to be influenced, at the margin, by cases having some easy symbolic tag like 'the baby in the drawer'. David Salt seemed to volunteer himself for the 'monster' label and the sheer number of health and welfare professionals who were involved was unusual. In most other respects, as far as the news values of the national press were concerned, the Charlene Salt trial was a routine case of provincial domestic misery, like that of Reuben Carthy.

Part of the press catechism is 'why?' If a child dies and outside agencies are involved, where does blame lie? Despite the political rejection of any collective obligation outside the family during the 1980s, there is no simple right/left cleavage in national press explanations of such situations. The Tory broadsheets are as interested in systems, policy, and politics as the *Guardian* and *The Independent*: hence the disjunction between the *Daily Telegraph*'s headline and text when it reported the Stephanie Fox inquiry report (21 June 1990). Political priorities and professional practice may be the target of criticism, but the search for guilty people is not a strong theme.

The focus on the individual is much more pervasive in the mid-market and mass tabloids. Here news framing practices and politics come together. We have seen the manifold reasons for refracting news through persons: doing so fulfils tabloid news values for both content and presentation. How do you make drama out of policy and process – or photograph it?

At the level of ideology, as we have seen in earlier chapters, this focus on the individual is a powerful two-edged weapon. First, the encompassing social and political system is rendered virtually invisible, and with it the very concept of systematic disadvantage, whether of class, gender, race, sexual orientation, age, disability, or any other socially constructed attribute.

Second, the radical right actively promulgates the model of society as merely an aggregate of autonomous individuals, personally responsible for their success or failure in the open market-place. As the law embodies individualism as moral responsibility, the notion that systems can bear 'blame' has been almost impossible to establish. Attempts, for example, to prove 'corporate manslaughter' have been notable by their failure. Social work public inquiries conducted by lawyers and set up along adversarial courtroom lines thus fit perfectly into the world view of the right-wing press generally, and into the news values of the tabloids particularly (Hallett 1989).

Were this not sufficient reason for newspapers like the *Daily Mail*, the *Daily Express*, the *Sun* and, in more diluted form, the *Daily Star* and *Today*, to hammer home the individualist message, they are dependent upon advertising for financial viability. Their readers must be wooed, not only to consume the paper for its news, features, etc., but as enthusiastic purchasers of the products advertised. These are overwhelmingly geared to lives based on private consumption in an introspective family-based household, or its equivalent. The *Sun*'s road to working-class liberation is hedonism in the private sphere, with (hetero)sexuality only as its most prominent manifestation.

In the autumn of 1992, when one piece of awful economic news was followed by another, the *Sun* turned savagely on the Major government. Even the miners became heroes – all miners, including members of the NUM. It has been suggested that this was primarily a craven demonstration of pseudo-independence by a Tory tabloid at a safe distance from an election. I would argue that this impetus was secondary; the main fount of the fury was the collapse of the implicit contract between Thatcher/Major Toryism and the section of the working class to which the *Sun* is crucially addressed.

In this sense, then, it is important to understand that social work and its vicissitudes are not singled out for vilification. It is rather that, in its intimate relationship with the family and the state, social services work offers a multi-faceted and very soft target for some sections of the national press when intervention seems to have failed in certain specific circumstances. Antithetically, there are other circumstances when any intervention at all is construed as a mistake, and still others when real mistakes seem not to produce the furore that they could have – or even should have.

Chapter 3

Abuse is alleged

A child dies; someone is convicted of her murder. In terms of guilt and violated rights the matter seems clear. The only disputed territory is whether the terrible event could have been prevented and, if so, by whom? If they did not, why not? The issues are stark and important, both of interest to the public and in the public interest. It is hardly surprising that trials for murder have always been a staple of the press. Fulfilling all their criteria of newsworthiness, they are one of the few topics that receive extended in-depth coverage by the mass tabloids.

For news media and for the wider public most of the time, the contest in court produces an outcome that is 'true'. The judicial process stands at the pinnacle of Becker's (1967) 'hierarchy of credibility'. After the verdict, other persons and interest groups can then join the hubbub over 'why did it happen?', perhaps taking the opportunity to pursue sectional interest, as Cohen (1973) describes in relation to the moral panic. Only if there is an appeal will serious questions be raised about the fit between the events recounted in court and 'reality'.

How, though, do the news media react when there is no agreement about events; where apparently reliable sources argue about how 'truth' should be discovered or understood; where there may be a conflict of civil rights? The first such instance, in County Cleveland in 1987, was the taking into care of a large number of children because medical examination had raised the possibility that they had been sexually abused. (See Cm 412 (1988), Illsley (1989), Nava (1988) and Parton (1991) for the events, subsequent public inquiry findings and media reaction.)

In this chapter the national press reports of three episodes will be examined: the events resulting from suspected ritual abuse in Rochdale; the uncovering of the 'pin-down' affair in Staffordshire; and the trial of Frank Beck for the sexual abuse of young people in residential care in Leicestershire.

SUSPICIONS OF RITUAL ABUSE IN ROCHDALE

In March 1990, four children from one family in Rochdale, Lancashire, were taken into care by Rochdale Social Services and made wards of court because of suspected ritual abuse. In June thirteen more children from the same area were made wards of court, of whom twelve were taken into care. Between June and September five children were returned to their parents, leaving twelve as wards of court. Three further children were taken into care in September. There was no news coverage of these events until early September, when intense pressure from media organizations, led by the *Mail on Sunday*, resulted in the modifying by a High Court judge of a blanket injunction which had restricted all public discussion of the case. In mid-September the Chief Constable of Greater Manchester announced that there would be no prosecutions, for lack of criminal evidence. The Rochdale Social Services Committee asked central government's Social Services Inspectorate to examine the department's practices; their report was received in October. After a High Court hearing lasting from December 1990 to March 1991 ten of the fifteen children still in care were returned home. The judgement, part of which was in open court, was very critical of some aspects of the social services department's work. Shortly afterwards the director of Rochdale Social Services resigned.

To compare and analyse the media coverage I have focused on certain key developments: the events of September 1990 (the lifting of the injunction, a further group of children taken into care, the statement by the Chief Constable, meetings of Rochdale Social Services); the SSI report of October 1990; the High Court judgement of March 1991; and the resignation of the director of social services.

The *Guardian*'s coverage of Rochdale started with three bylined articles on p. 2. Both the amount of detail and the format immediately signal that this is a complex issue with several discrete dimensions of interest to readers. The first is headed 'Parents and council battle over children' under the ambiguous strapline 'Judge removes gag on 17 taken into care in abuse case' (10 September 1990). It sketches the events to date in neutral hard news format, interweaving the substance of the allegations with the media law issues. The second item reviews the controversy over the extent or even existence of ritual abuse. Experts on both sides are quoted but the phrase 'little firm evidence' in the standfirst implies a sceptical authorial and/or editorial eye. In the third, slightly shorter piece, the paper's legal correspondent cites prominent legal voices to explain the 'ban on publishing'.

The next day the bylined story led p. 3: 'Satanic abuse total grows' (*Guardian* 11 September 1990). The contested nature of the issue is clear from the presentation, which both describes events and reproduces claims from parents and the social services department. The following day (12 September) a story at the top of p. 6 further underlined the complexity of the dispute, reporting that a local councillor who was a member of the social services committee was trying to prevent the taking of wardship proceedings because of the limitation on information entailed. BASW is quoted as the balancing voice against this course of action.

On 13 September the *Guardian*'s second news page was dominated by a large picture of the Rochdale estate concerned, above two articles. The first reported the demands of PAIN (Parents Against Injustice) that the DoH should become involved. No social work or council spokesperson is quoted; there is also an update on events. A second and almost equally long item is very much the 'colour' story about how much the residents of the estate at the centre of the affair resent their notoriety. It foregrounds their utter scepticism, using sources who are clearly meant to be credible: clergy and salt-of-the-earth locals.

Further complexity was introduced in a p. 3 hard news article on the day after, headlined 'Police drop satanic ritual abuse cases' (*Guardian* 14 September 1990). The police statement in fact refers to some charges against some people in a variety of localities. The item also reports councillor/professional staff conflict, further legal difficulties and finishes with an expert in support of the credence given by the social workers to children's evidence. A second leader on 14 September suggests that 'Rochdale could launch a serious examination of ritual abuse' and that 'Judgements in the Rochdale case should be suspended until more facts have been tested'. The writer points out that although the more dramatic warnings of fundamentalist Christians about the extent of ritual abuse have not been substantiated, 'it is silly to pretend there is no evidence of ritual abuse' – although the leader writer does not bring forward any evidence to support this assertion.

On Saturday, 10 November, the *Guardian* asserted, on p. 3, 'Ritual abuse cases "were mishandled"', and continues with a version of the as-yet-unreleased SSI report from the *Manchester Evening News* (the *Guardian*'s sister paper), together with a denial from Rochdale council. When the SSI report actually appeared, the paper gave it moderate prominence on its second news page. The second paragraph concludes: 'the report is not notably critical, contrary to advance speculation' (13 November 1990) – but does not mention its own credulity. In the story the key SSI findings are interspersed with news of its reception by the health minister and comment from the Family Rights Group. That day the *Guardian* also discussed the issues in a second leader. The strong message is that the SSI report is 'a relatively clean sheet', in the SSI's own terms. Most of the rest of the article is directed at calls for national guidance on a number of key aspects of practice – typical professional concerns of the readership. But, as the *Guardian* says, 'So what prompted the weekend reports of a pending denunciation?' and answers itself 'It looks like media manipulation by leakers intent on pushing the "stolen children" line.' This hints at the extent of pressure group activity in this and similar cases, and also embodies an assumption of media autonomy in ironic contrast to subsequent changes of orientation.

The *Guardian*'s coverage thus far, while sympathetic to the political environment and to the claims of the parents, had been framed within professional discourse – as one would expect from its market. Even scepticism about ritual abuse is treated as being a matter also of professional debate. When, however, the High Court judgement both overturned and comprehensively criticized the social services department's actions, the *Guardian* embraced the new perspective completely. On 8 March 1991 most of p. 2 was given over to four articles with two pictures: 'Rochdale children returned to parents'. A white-on-black strapline 'Judge rules out satanic abuse claims; Social services department breached guidelines; Council evidence "seriously misleading"', together with a large picture of an aggrieved parent and a smaller one of the judge, rams home where the problem now lies. One of the articles summarizes the judgement; another quotes legal experts describing the criticism of social services as 'unprecedented'. A further colour piece describes the effects of the affair on local residents. Another repeats, without comment, some of the children's accounts which had originally triggered the case. As it follows the judge's castigation of the work (although not of the workers' intentions), especially their methods of eliciting and recording evidence, presumably the inferential framework is that only those with a predisposition to do so would have taken the stories literally.

The *Guardian* is not pulling its punches. The first leader that day is headed 'Rochdale: simply a terrible botch' and opens 'Just because you feel a scapegoat doesn't mean you are not at fault' (8 March 1991). Apart from a brief obeisance to the difficulty of social work in the final paragraph, the text focuses on the children's suffering, in the context of complete acceptance of the judgement. It is treated not only as demonstrating that the social services had failed to produce any evidence to support their action in most (but not all) of the cases, but that there had been no abuse. There is no reference to those instances of ritual abuse used in the 14 September 1991 editorial to support its argument that the issue was the nature and extent of ritual abuse, rather than its reality.

On 9 March 'Abuse case head quits' (*Guardian*) led p. 3. The news item contains an account of events together with local reactions of regret and is bracketed with a colour piece on the '"Decent bloke" caught in satanic tangle'. In this the director is characterized as 'tragically caught between demands for the safety of children, the rights of parents to look after their own children, unnerving stories of satanic rituals and a lack of adequate financial resources'. This, and the rest of the item in the same tone, makes a curious contrast with the harsh, unequivocal, somewhat oversimplified – and very un-*Guardian*-like – leader of the previous day.

The first news of the Rochdale events appeared in the *Daily Telegraph* on 8 September 1990, immediately following the relaxation of the injunction the previous day. The bylined story, at the top of p. 3, although opened and closed with the official framework, is popular rather than professional-aligned. Most of the text is given to the experiences of one of the parents involved, together with the complaint by local Childwatch 'that the case was a "travesty of the parents' basic rights"'. On 11 September, the *Daily Telegraph* followed up with a brief unbylined and descriptive item on p. 3 reporting 'More children removed in Satanic abuse investigation'. Two days later another short piece on p. 2 mentioned Rochdale in the context of a case in neighbouring Manchester. On p. 21, however, there was a large feature, 'A town's talk of the devil' (*Daily Telegraph* 13 September 1990), illustrated with a dramatic picture juxtaposing bleak blocks of flats with a graveyard crucifix and a smaller montage of lurid newspaper headlines. The text is notable for the even-handedness with which it sets out the complexity of the issues. Aggrieved parents, incredulous residents of the estate, and disgruntled councillors are offset by the 'appalling dilemma' of the social workers. The yet greater difficulties in gaining evidence than in Cleveland are made clear: 'the Rochdale case is floating in deeper waters – and they don't come much deeper than what goes on in a child's head', but then the possibility is raised that workers in the case had been over-influenced by NSPCC publicity given to the problem of ritual abuse. A councillor complains about the parents' powerlessness; the author suggests that small children 'only' watching horror videos could well be considered 'reason enough for the social services' concern', and follows this with a bit of investigative work about the trade in bootleg video nasties on the estate.

On 15 September a straight news item on p. 5 headed 'Council staff in child abuse case backed' reported the social services committee's actions without 'balancing' comment from any other party.

Like the *Guardian*, the *Daily Telegraph* gave space to the leaked account of the SSI report in November, again in hard news format on p. 7 (10 November). The account of the actual report (13 November) was equally neutral.

The *Daily Telegraph* made the High Court ruling its p. 1 lead: '"Satanic ritual abuse" children freed by judge' was followed by a long and very detailed account (three and a half full columns) on p. 2. This was bylined 'Press Association', setting it within the framework of legal affairs, rather than professional debate or popular human interest. Most of the p. 1 story was also taken up with the content of the judgement, with brief comment from the department, a councillor, and the solicitor for one of the families. Clearly the *Telegraph*, like the *Guardian*, regarded the judgement as axiomatically resolving the issue: the use of 'freed' and the distancing quotation marks around 'Satanic ritual abuse' in the headline are an implicit acceptance of the blameworthiness of the social services, despite the neutrality of the text. A first leader on the same day (8 March 1991) is trenchant: the events were 'extraordinary and horrible'; the interviews with children were conducted 'incompetently'; the social workers are characterized as ill-educated.

> What happened ... was that people with the legal power to take children away from their families were so possessed by an idea that they ignored the requirements of evidence, or proper procedure, and, it must be said, of ordinary human decency.
>
> (*Daily Telegraph* 8 March 1991)

In keeping with the paper's right-wing philosophy the writer is indignant that the social workers involved have been able to stay anonymous. But, interestingly, there is no invocation of idealized 'family values'. One of the concluding observations is that the preoccupation with ritual abuse is 'hampering the investigation of that more mundane but almost equally vile abuse of children that does take place'.

The willingness of the *Telegraph* to keep complexity in view was confirmed on 9 September. On p. 1 a small news item reported the resignation of the director, together with the DoH-sponsored research review of ritual abuse. Page 13 is dominated by a feature interview with the director of the NSPCC, who, lest we think him a wet liberal, is described as a 'former chief probation officer ... hardened to the front-line realities of crime and social deviance'. The substance of the article is entirely given to his point of view, not even mentioning that the NSPCC was directly involved in the Rochdale events and the subject of criticism. He is quoted as rejecting the possibility that the NSPCC has manufactured a problem where none exists, pointing out the vital requirement '"to differentiate between *evidential* and *therapeutic* needs"' in practice (emphasis in original), and his fear that the issue will turn into a '"battle between the rights of children and the rights of parents"'. Significantly, although the *Daily Telegraph* seemed poised to frame the events in these terms at the outset, its later coverage moved away from this template, unlike the right-wing tabloids.

The first reports of the events in Rochdale did not appear in the *Daily Mail* until 13 September 1990, despite the central role played in the legal controversy by its sister paper the *Mail on Sunday*. A large article on p. 17 embodies disbelief in its presentation: '33 children in "satanic rites" probe'. Even at this early stage the second paragraph reads 'The investigations centre on whether the children were emotionally or sexually abused during bizarre and depraved occult rituals, or whether their chilling stories are fantasies fuelled by watching video nasties'. Social services, although quoted at some length, are constructed as defending themselves against this explanation for their 'swoops' on homes. The story closes with a parent saying the affair was all a mistake.

The *Mail*'s rejection of the social services' position was even clearer the next day in a very large headline on p. 2: '"Satan case" parents in clear, say police'. The opening sections reproduce elements of the Chief Constable's statement, without any qualifying material to make the distinction between the inability to collect criminal evidence and what might nevertheless have occurred. A third of the text is devoted, without an offsetting voice, to a local councillor wholly in support of the parents: '"It has all been a horrendous mistake. The excuse that officials have been hiding behind ... The children were never involved in witchcraft or Satanism."' Further down, the phrase 'had claimed' is applied to the director of social services, giving a clear signal of his place in the 'hierarchy of credibility'.

The *Daily Mail* did not need SSI reports or High Court judgements to come to a conclusion about the issues. On 15 September it devoted its leader column to the 'Lost children of Rochdale'. While social workers 'Of course' are 'in an unenviable situation' and 'Obviously parents should not allow six-year olds to watch sadistic videos', social workers should not 'grab' and 'institutionalize' children because they have become 'over-zealous, preferring the superiority of their ideological preconceptions to either the views of the police or any evidence to the contrary ... Such awesome power would be the envy of many a totalitarian state.' The rest of the page is filled with a feature 'Death of a satanic myth', with the strapline 'IS THERE A SINGLE SHRED OF REAL EVIDENCE TO SHOW A CULT OF DEVIL WORSHIP?' The article, which originally appeared in the *Independent on Sunday*, takes the line that there is no evidence of widespread satanism, in the UK or elsewhere. Rather it is to be explained as an outcome of local mass hysteria coupled with the modern 'social problems' industry, promulgated in the US by a '"loose network" of therapists, fundamentalist Christians, serving and ex-police officers and ... the media'. UK experience is then adduced to support this thesis.

When accounts of the SSI report were circulated before its release, the *Daily Mail* asserted that it 'had a copy of the draft 46-page report of the Social Services Inspectorate, which was called for by [the] Health Minister' (*Daily Mail* 10 November 1990). This formed the basis of its p. 1 splash '"SATAN" COUNCIL CONDEMNED' – an interesting lexical juxtaposition. Most of the story reproduces points from the report, described by the *Guardian* as 'a relatively clean sheet', as we have seen. That the report was, for legal reasons, about practice in general based on other cases is mentioned only in passing. So too is the fact that the report was not instigated by the minister but was the outcome of a request to her by the council itself. This disjunction between paragraphs four and eleven is made easier to sustain by the *Mail*'s not having reported the September meeting of the Rochdale Social Services Committee which had, albeit with reservations, backed its professional staff. Bracketed with the p. 2 report is a box headed 'All we want is our children back', quoting two couples involved and a solicitor for four families. 'However, council chiefs ... stood by what they had done' (*Daily Mail* 10 November 1990).

The formal publication of the report, described as 'exclusively revealed' in the *Daily Mail*, was covered on p. 21, under the large headline 'A parent's right to know', with the white-on-black strapline 'GOVERNMENT ATTACKS ROCHDALE IN CHILD ABUSE CONTROVERSY' and standfirst 'Lessons of Cleveland must be learned, says Mrs Bottomley' (*Daily Mail* 13 November 1990). The story begins, 'Health Minister Virginia Bottomley yesterday joined in the criticism of the council at the centre of the "satanic" abuse controversy'. In a closing paragraph the director is described as having said procedures would be 'brought up to scratch', a usage which implies that this is a straightforward matter which need never have arisen. The article report is bracketed with a story that Rochdale councillors have 'rallied around' a (pictured) councillor over a conviction for a sexual offence against an adult, nine years before, at the other end of the country.

As might be expected, the High Court judgement filled most of p. 1 of the *Daily Mail*: 'BACK WITH THEIR FAMILIES' under the strapline 'Snatched children can go home says judge' (8 March 1991). Although technically a hard news item, allegations 'haunted', the judge 'demolished' and parents 'wept'. It continued inside, where the case filled p. 5. Grouped around the large headline 'End of the nightmare' are five further stories and a picture of the solicitor representing some of the parents. Two short items point up parallels with the Orkney events and the role of the *Mail on Sunday* in the 'legal battle'. In another pair 'Judge points out the way to safety' was placed beside 'We will do better, says welfare chief', calling up the image of a naughty boy summoned before a firm but kind headmaster. In fact the 'welfare chief' is only given space to assure the minister that 'his department will pull its socks up' – another banal and demeaning image. The privileged voices are the judge, the minister, the solicitor – and the parents: 'My Mother's Day gift: A thousand hugs and kisses'.

The same edition contains a savage first leader, about social workers' 'almost untrammelled power' enabling them to repeat 'the kind of scandalous oppression of innocent parents in Cleveland' (*Daily Mail* 8 March 1991) 'Oppression' is a word popular on the left, but used by the right only in relation to alien regimes. The injunctions banning publicity are characterized as 'an attempt to cover up the social workers' catastrophic blunder', which seems a difficult conclusion to draw as the injunctions dated from the first wardship proceedings, rather than when widespread doubts started to be expressed. The editorial concludes 'But it remains a disgrace to a country like ours which takes pride in its long tradition of personal freedom that social workers can with so little justification still trample on such rights with such ease'. (The rest of the page is given to 'A very rotten borough', a feature on 'Tirana-on-Thames, more commonly known as Lambeth', which apparently had Trotskyites on the council.)

On 9 September the *Daily Mail* reported the resignation of the director of social services. Although the regret of colleagues is included, it is offset by an unattributed claim that he 'jumped before he was pushed'. His support for his professional staff is portrayed as having 'backed the women's case, despite mounting disbelief'.

In its initial treatment of the Rochdale story, the *Sun* took very much the same line as the *Daily Mail*, although expressed in its distinctive idiom with a large headline leading p. 5: '17 CHILDREN SEIZED IN SATAN SEX CULT RAIDS'; 'Boy "saw babes killed"'(8 September 1990). 'Social workers have snatched 17 kids from their parents in a Satanic sex abuse scare . . . But NO charges have been brought . . . And they say the scare is the result of one little boy's FANTASIES after watching video nasties.' The bylined article goes on to quote parents, their supporters and the police, but not social services. On 11 September 'Fear over devil gag on kiddies' was a brief item by the same journalist explaining that parents were being denied access to their children for fear that they might 'use devil cult words or symbols to silence victims'. The children had been 'rounded up'; the parents were 'distraught'. Two days later the *Sun* mentioned the Rochdale events in a neutral descriptive item on p. 15, reporting the statement by the Chief Constable of Manchester.

The distinctive *Sun* inflection on the SSI report was to make it the final paragraph of 'SORDID PAST OF GAY REV IN SATAN KIDS ROW' (13 November 1990). Most of the 22 column cm on p. 5 recount the 'gay rev's' personal details and the alleged Tory/Labour split over the matter.

The High Court judgement in March 1991 was grouped with the director's resignation in a small descriptive piece at the foot of p. 2, concluding 'Mr Justice Douglas Brown returned 10 children to their parents on Thursday. He branded social workers "amateurish" for believing kids' tales of abuse' (*Sun* 9 March 1991). There was no editorial follow-up.

The *Daily Mirror* gave the early phases of the Rochdale events very brief coverage, perhaps because considerable space was occupied with the campaign of the then proprietor, the late Robert Maxwell, against the president of the National Union of Mineworkers, Arthur Scargill. The first mention, on 14 September 1990, is at the foot of p. 5: 'Satan probe ditched', neutrally reporting the Chief Constable's announcement that there were to be no criminal prosecutions. The next day (15 September) a short item on p. 7, 'Clash on Satanic sex kids', set the claims of the social services against those of the parents in descriptive hard news format.

As in the *Sun*, *Daily Mirror* readers were alerted to the professional advice of the SSI below the headline 'Devil-kids Rev's "gay sex" case' (13 November 1990). The brief p. 7 story starts with three paragraphs on the 'row' and then continues that 'Whitehall watchdogs' had 'slammed the council', before concluding with a councillor's defence of his gay colleague.

The *Daily Mirror* abruptly changed pitch when the High Court judgement appeared, making it a p. 1 splash on 8 March: 'HOME!' (in 4.5 cm type); 'Social workers lashed as "Satan kids" are set free'. The front page article lists some of the 'gross series of blunders' and the story continues over the whole of p. 5 headed 'THEY EVEN BANNED XMAS CARDS FROM MUM AND DAD' with the inset headline 'We have been to hell and back. Our lives just crumbled'. The dramatic presentation, credited to three journalists, is illustrated with small pictures of the director of social services and the health minister and a larger, but uncaptioned, picture of a man with two small children walking, head down, away from the camera on a run-down estate. The main text summarizes the background and some of the main points of the judgement. Smaller items are headed 'Shamed leader accepts verdict' and 'DAWN RAIDS RAPPED' by the minister, who is, however, quoted as saying that social workers 'faced a dilemma'. BASW is briefly quoted as a professional response to the judge's recommendations. In the same edition, the *Daily Mirror* made an editorial comment, condemning Rochdale Social Services for poor practice. It concludes that such episodes risk discouraging people from acting on their suspicions of 'real and terrible abuse of children', but does not commit itself to the non-existence of ritual abuse.

On 9 March the *Daily Mirror* reported the resignation of the director in standard hard news format on p. 7.

THE CONDEMNATION OF PIN-DOWN

In June 1990 a television documentary gave the first national publicity to the technique of controlling children in some Staffordshire children's homes known as 'pin-down'. The technique, originated in 1983 by local residential workers Tony Latham and (secondarily) Phil Price, did not use physical force, but was based on the principles of behaviour modification. Children who were alleged to have misbehaved were deprived of 'privileges'; in extreme cases this consisted of being confined to a sparsely furnished room in night clothes for long periods. The practice, which was never concealed, continued until 1989 when a local solicitor took wardship proceedings on behalf of two residents. An independent investigation by Allan Levy QC and Barbara Kahan was set up by the social services committee in July 1990; they reported in May 1991 (Levy and Kahan 1991). The most important aspect of pin-down was the emotional damage to the young people involved, for which Staffordshire has since paid compensation. Staff have been dismissed, but no criminal charges have been laid.

There were, however, a number of other aspects to the affair. The most significant was a network of enterprises under the umbrella name Fundwell, set up from the mid-1970s by Tony Latham, financed by government training initiatives, and staffed by young people in care. Questions were raised about whether these were training or punishment, and about the propriety of placing council contracts with Fundwell. Yet further dimensions included: officer/elected member failures of communication and accountability; party-political disputes; the failure of the SSI to detect and end the practice; rumours of Masonic links; questions about visits by known paedophiles to some residents.

Apart from its intrinsic importance, the controversy about pin-down marked the start of a series of revelations about the abuse of power in residential care throughout the UK, raising questions in turn about children's rights; social services resources, management and priorities; government policies; and the training, pay and recruitment of residential child care staff.

National press coverage for two key periods in the controversy over pin-down was examined: first, the broadcasting of the documentary; second, the period from just before the publication of the Levy/Kahan report at the end of May 1991 through to the end of June 1991.

The television revelations were broadcast on 25 June 1990. None of the newspapers sampled (the *Guardian*; the *Daily Telegraph*; the *Daily Mail*; the *Sun* and the *Daily Mirror*) mentioned the issue at all on 25, 26 or 27 June. This is surprising, since not only do news media make extensive use of other media as cheap sources of material, but documentaries are often given advance publicity by news release or even linked newspaper features. It may be that coverage was planned, but swamped by the IRA bombing of a well-known London club with strong Conservative Party links on the evening of 25 June.

The Levy/Kahan report was formally published on 31 May 1991. Coverage in *The Independent* was very extensive indeed, and set in a much larger context. On 27 May there had been a p. 1 lead and the whole of p. 3 on alleged ill-treatment at Ty Mawr, a children's home in Gwent. The first leader that day was headed 'Children's homes that don't care'. Although it talks of 'foolish or wicked behaviour by staff', the editorial locates the problem at the policy level: lack of central direction and funding, leading to poor local control, and a lack of skills and unattractive job prospects in residential social work. The same issue was the p. 1 lead again on 29 May: 'Children's homes inquiry ordered', with the strapline 'Minister demands action to end abuses, but social service chiefs ask where the money is coming from'. In the text two further homes are mentioned; a report on one, in Norfolk, fills p. 3.

On 30 May another p. 1 item grouped Ty Mawr with predictions about the general content of the Levy/Kahan report, highlighting failures of management and of the SSI. The Secretary of State is quoted, as are critical comments from Barnardo's.

The actual publication of the report was given the p. 1 lead, the whole of pp. 2 and 3, a leader, and a supporting feature, signalling an issue of great importance. The front page is headed 'Pin-down victims to seek damages' (*The Independent* 31 May 1991) with a secondary item 'Human rights violated report says', briefly summarizing the findings. For a broadsheet, the treatment is highly emotive. There is a picture of a young man who had experienced the regime with his arm around Barbara Kahan. A cartoon of a butterfly being stuck with a pin is inset into the first lead, beside highlighted recommendations. The main text cites a wide range of interested parties: the report's authors; representatives of residents; central government; the SSI; local politicians; Tony Latham.

Inside, the two main news pages are devoted to an elaborate presentation of the issues with nine separate items and four photographs: of the report's authors; of one of the homes; of the chair of social services; of Tony Latham. The organizing theme is the usual policy and politics focus of the national broadsheets, with a long article summarizing the findings of the report headed 'Senior managers blamed for inhumane practices'. The same interpretation follows under 'Authorities ignored warnings on regime', which recounts the report's findings and the recriminations between politicians and officers in Staffordshire about who knew what and when. 'Human interest' is again given unusual prominence. The personal details of Levy and Kahan and of Latham are described, and two harrowing 'case studies' of residents' experiences presented. Two subsidiary articles by medical correspondents explore the damage caused by pin-down and the weakness of health provision for young people in care.

In a first leader, *The Independent* constructs the problem as system failure. 'Residential care has become a Cinderella service' (*The Independent* 31 May 1991) needing better trained front-line staff, 'adequate protection for whistleblowers' and an 'independent and pro-active inspectorate'. On the facing page is an interview with the current chief inspector. The title – 'However did this happen?' – and tone is mildly aggressive, as 'Sir Bill is in the hot seat' having to explain that his staff picked up no hint of pin-down. 'As they did not know of its existence they were not empowered to carry out an inspection: a problem must first be identified to trigger the procedure.' Below is a case history by Masud Hoghughi, director of a centre for 'disordered adolescents', reinforcing the argument that residential work is undervalued. Even the paper's main cartoon is about pin-down. It shows a child pinned beneath a heap of crushed public-sector functionaries.

On 1 June *The Independent* gave prominent p. 2 coverage to

developments over Ty Mawr and another parallel case in Scotland. The paper's heavy investment in the issue is indicated by references in the articles to its own role in fuelling public debate. Further news of Ty Mawr and of central government action on Scottish children's homes appeared on p. 2 on 5 June, bracketed with developments over the Orkney child abuse events. On 18 June *The Independent* mentioned pin-down in the last paragraph of a p. 2 item on the use of drugs to control young people in a Dorset children's home. Again on 24 June pin-down was mentioned in a round-up of related items closing another p. 2 story about the charges to be laid against Frank Beck (see below). The final news item on residential care in the study period appeared on 26 June 1991, when the Dorset case was again reported, linked to a similar case at the St Charles Youth Treatment Centre in Essex.

The *Daily Telegraph*'s coverage was mainly focused on pin-down and did not give detailed attention to similar instances. The first report (30 May 1991) was a bylined news item on p. 3 previewing the Levy/Kahan report. The issues are framed as political/professional; in the opening paragraph it is stated that the report is 'seen by ministers as of equal importance to the 1988 Cleveland inquiry into child abuse'. The whole emphasis is on the failure of systems, with no mention of the individual workers nor of related questions about Fundwell. Brief details of the report are interwoven with expected action from the minister, questions about the SSI, and staffing changes in Staffordshire. The final paragraphs draw attention to moves towards foster care, and the low proportion of qualified staff in residential social work, with the last word coming from the NSPCC, calling on the government to make residential care higher priority.

On 31 May pin-down was the second lead on p. 1 of the *Telegraph*, with 'Pindown wrong, admits creator' above a short summary of the issue, both topped by a large version of the picture of Barbara Kahan and a former 'pindown child'. The whole of p. 2 is devoted to pin-down and problems with residential child care elsewhere, with six articles and three pictures, the largest of another former resident, who gives a brief account of her experiences. The organizing theme is that pin-down was an utterly open and well-intentioned idea which went unchecked because child care was underdeveloped and under-resourced in Staffordshire. The summary of Tony Latham's part in the affair, far from attributing personal blame, stresses that local management knew and approved of his methods. (Perhaps there is a touch of relish in the reproduction of inquiry evidence that Labour-controlled Staffordshire was '"in a time-warp"' with an '"inward-looking culture"' (*Daily Telegraph* 31 May 1991)). This frame is reinforced in a p. 17 feature: 'The world of Tony Latham, where child care is just a poor relation'. The standfirst runs 'With little formal training, they have to look after the most disturbed children. [Bylined author] explains how a residential child care home could go so wrong.' The text uses a number of senior professionals and BASW to set out the residual nature of contemporary residential care, the low proportion of qualified staff, difficulties of finding an effective regime, poor pay and prospects, etc.

'The wider responsibility' for pin-down was the subject of the second leader (*Daily Telegraph* 31 May 1991). Although it opens with a round condemnation of Staffordshire, it locates the problem firmly in the social structure: in 'an intensely self-centred society . . . there is amongst us a growing proportion of children who can only be described as feral' who cause problems for the police and for schools. It concludes 'We shall not reduce their numbers by placing sole blame and responsibility upon social workers'. There is no proposed solution; changes in family patterns are not mentioned, perhaps surprisingly for a paper seen as traditional Tory.

The next mention in the *Daily Telegraph* came in an item on 1 June: '"Pindown" staff may face sack'. This neutral hard news story on p. 4 describes the procedures in hand to discipline a wide range of council employees criticized in the inquiry report. It concludes with the 'renewed call' of the local Conservative MP for the resignation of the Labour chair of Staffordshire Social Services. The issue continued to be refracted through the political lens when, on 3 June, a p. 4 report covered the minister's forthcoming Commons statement on pin-down and 'new and stringent requirements for children's homes'. The story, credited to the Press Association, is based on an interview the previous day, at which the minister (who is pictured) made her much-repeated call for '"street-wise grannies" back in children's homes'. (The full context suggests, however, that the intention was that they should be qualified and employed, rather than this being yet another variation on the 'anyone can do social work' theme.) A shorter story below gathers together the setting up of helplines, problems at other homes, and the SSI denial that it had 'failed to recognize pindown'.

Residential child care in Scotland and Wales was raised again by the *Telegraph* on 5 June in a p. 4 news item, bylined 'Scottish Correspondent'. On 6 June a 'Health Services Correspondent' summarizes Tony Latham's defence of his work in a *Social Work Today* interview, without quoting a contradicting source. Coverage continued on 8 June in relation to Coventry, on p. 6 bylined 'Social Services Correspondent'. The local politics of the issue reappeared on 14 June when the Staffordshire Social

Services Committee's vote of confidence in the chair was reported on p. 4 within the framework of continuing mutual accusations between him, the county council Conservative group, and a local Labour MP, again in stand-ard for-and-against news format. On 25 June the misuse of drugs by staff at the St Charles Youth Treatment Centre was prominently reported on p. 2, together with one paragraph on the Dorset case. This account, though bylined 'Health Services Correspondent', was triggered by the Secretary of State's response to two reports, by DoH inspectors and the SSI.

Like *The Independent*, the *Daily Mail* started reporting pin-down in advance of the appearance of the Levy/Kahan report. 'Victory in sight for council's locked-in children' (*Daily Mail* 27 May 1991) was the headline over a p. 9 report that began

> All day, every day, [a pensioner couple] saw and heard the suffering of the children held in solitary confinement at a council home opposite their flat. Sometimes the tearful, half-naked youngsters held up signs begging: 'Phone my mum and get me out'.
>
> (*Daily Mail* 27 May 1991)

The report goes on to say that 'None of the children had committed any crimes' and to anticipate 'the report of an inquiry headed by Mr Allen Levy QC' [*sic*]. (By the next day the *Daily Mail* was still talking of the 'Levy report' and using the construction 'says barrister Allan Levy', but now he chaired the inquiry 'with child care expert Barbara Kahan'. Is it that the *Daily Mail* has difficulty recognizing women experts, or that 'child care expert' is an oxymoron for the paper?) More details of the regime and staff involved are included and a resident is quoted.

The contents of the inquiry were the p. 1 lead: 'NOT AGAIN!; Children in care were locked away for months' with the strapline 'Another scandal faces social services'. It opens: 'The tarnished reputation of Britain's social workers is stained by yet another scandal today' (*Daily Mail* 30 May 1991). The text consists mainly of a précis of the report and continues on to p. 2 headed 'Pindown scandal'. The secretary of the ADSS 'denied the problems in Staffordshire were being repeated elsewhere'; action by the minister and the SSI is briefly mentioned. Within the news story is a large inset box containing two pictures (of Tony Latham and of one of the homes) and two further stories. One recounts how 'The legacy of pindown still haunts' a former resident. The other item lists 'TEN WHO ARE NAMED IN THE REPORT'. This placing of individuals in the foreground implies that they should be held entirely and personally responsible for the events – an interpretation reinforced by the omission of the local political background.

Despite the prominence given to the pin-down issue and the clear interpretative framework imposed, the p. 1 lead is bylined 'Daily Mail Reporter', which implies few resources had been deployed to obtain specialized background or fresh angles. This did not prevent a sweeping editorial condemnation in the *Daily Mail* on 30 May: 'Yet another official report roundly criticises social workers . . . This time it concerns homes run by the Socialist Staffordshire County Council where children were subjected to a harsh, illegal punishment known as "pindown".' The writer goes on to reject the notion that lack of money is the root cause, but asserts that it is 'yet another example' of local government bureaucratic routines.

'"Children's homes need grannies to help"' (*Daily Mail* 3 June 1991) headed p. 15 and is a straight account of the Press Association interview with the minister. On 4 June an article, on p. 6 without byline, gathered together the minister's calls for local authority checks on homes, the setting up of helplines, criticisms of Staffordshire, action by the SSI and opposition comment on residential care. An editorial on the same day was scathing:

> It has become almost routine every time there is an official inquiry into some resounding failure by social workers to fulfil their duty . . . for no disciplinary action to be taken . . . all those in Staffordshire who are culpable in any way must either resign or be sacked.
>
> (*Daily Mail* 4 June 1991)

At the end of June the St Charles furore was given high-profile treatment, leading p. 1, continued on to p. 2 and as the subject of the first leader (*Daily Mail* 25 June 1991). The report, attributed to a 'Medical Correspondent', is largely based on two official reports and the Secretary of State's response to them. The concluding paragraphs name the suspended director, who was 'unavailable for comment', and refer to the pin-down policy. In its editorial comment the *Mail* underlines the challenging behaviour of the young people at the 'Government-run' centre but asserts 'Children who become hard cases do not forfeit their rights as human beings.' The leader writer's worries are, though, mitigated by the success of the regime at Glenthorne, 'the only other centre of its kind in the land', presumably on the strength of the SSI report.

When the Levy/Kahan report appeared, the *Daily Mirror* gave it full-scale tabloid treatment: the whole of pp. 1, 4 and 5, plus editorial comment (30 May 1991). The front page is headlined 'HOW COULD IT HAPPEN?' as a subscript to pictures of Tony Latham and one of the homes with the dramatic caption (1 cm type in white-on-black) 'Inside this council home this social worker organised a regime of terror, torment, humiliation and solitary confinement for children as young as nine. Yet nobody did anything for SIX YEARS.' The continuation forms part of a double page spread under the banner headline (in 3 cm type and white-on-black) 'PLEASE PHONE MY MUM AND TELL HER TO GET ME OUT OF HERE; Neighbours saw the pindown kids' despair'. Most of the text tells the harrowing story of residents; the Fundwell dimension is briefly mentioned towards the end, as are central and local government responses. A small bylined article raises another dimension: 'SEX PERVERT VISITED HOMES'.

As in other papers, the human and dramatic aspects of the affair are underlined with pictures: a large one of Tony Latham; three small shots of 'HELL HOMES'. Unlike other papers, the *Mirror* also has pictures of two named ex-residents and adds an artist's impression of a desolate child in a 'pindown room'. Despite the foregrounding of the personal, however, the *Daily Mirror* does not explain the events in wholly individual terms. The report 'lays the bulk of the blame at the feet of Mr Latham. But . . . it was shared by senior and middle management in Staffordshire's social services department.' This is also the line taken in the editorial comment, where a highlighted sentence reads 'How could monitoring of the homes have been so lax? Or the authorities so fooled?' It then mentions problems and allegations elsewhere, and advocates fostering as both easier to 'police' and cheaper.

On 31 May the *Daily Mirror* gave the case an even bigger headline. In 4 cm type, the words themselves took a third of the front page: 'PINDOWN: WHY I DID IT; "It was aversion therapy so that children would want to go home"'. Tony Latham is now centre-stage, described as 'defiant' and 'disgraced' in his 'amazing attempt to justify' pin-down – in fact a statement made through his lawyers. The report continues on p. 2, where Fundwell is briefly introduced, juxtaposed with mentions of his home, family and salary. The publication of the Levy/Kahan report is summarized as '"IT MUST NEVER HAPPEN AGAIN"' – a quotation from Allan Levy, who is pictured. In the *Mirror*'s version, Barbara Kahan also features as an 'expert'. A reply from social services and further allegations from the National Association for Young People in Care (NAYPIC) concluded the story.

Despite the opprobrium heaped on Tony Latham individually, the *Daily Mirror* persists in an attempt to put the case in a wider context. The whole of the top half of p. 2 is devoted to a very lengthy (by its usual presentational conventions) editorial comment headed 'Throwaway people'. The argument is that the line of responsibility for pin-down branches out from specific people who should have done something –

doctors, teachers, inspectors, neighbours – to the whole national political culture in which poverty, selfishness and a premium on winning flourish. Social workers are to blame only to the extent that they are 'unenlightened, untrained', 'the cheap labour of a civilised society'. The leader writer's conclusion is that the 'Staffordshire scandal' may yield some good if we 'face up to the fact that children in care are not born to be uncontrollable. They . . . are because we have made them so.'

On 1 June the *Mirror* reported complaints about the regime at two other children's homes, signalled as continuing news by an inset picture of an earlier front page. 'PINDOWN FURY' (*Daily Mirror* 3 June 1991) headed the brief account of the health minister's call for 'streetwise grannies'. She is also quoted as saying that the local authority 'singularly failed in its duty'.

The only other mention of pin-down and related issues by the *Daily Mirror* was a very short item on 26 June 1991 about the Dorset home case.

The *Sun* (30 May) reported the publication of the Levy/Kahan report with five neutral one-sentence paragraphs on p. 2; the only other mention of residential child care in the *Sun* during the period scrutinized was on 25 June 1991. Lacking a sexual angle on the misuse of drugs on residents at St Charles Youth Treatment Centre, the paper uses another favourite template: war games. 'SCANDAL SQUAD RAIDERS BOOT OUT HOME BOSS' introduced the p. 11 story of the Secretary of State's 'secret operation' in which a 'Welfare squad swooped', while the minister 'waited by the phone'. The link with pin-down is mentioned in the last paragraph.

THE FRANK BECK CASE

In a case lasting ten weeks between mid-September and the end of November 1991, Frank Beck was tried, with two co-defendants, at Leicester Crown Court. Frank Beck pleaded not guilty to all sixty charges against him. The prosecution did not proceed with thirty-three of the charges. On one other count the judge discharged the jury from reaching a verdict. Frank Beck was acquitted of nine charges, but found guilty of the remaining seventeen. He was sentenced to five life sentences for rape and buggery and to twenty-four years for buggery, attempted buggery, indecent assault, and actual bodily harm, the sentences to run concurrently. Most of the charges related to young people resident in the homes under Beck's control, the rest to male social work staff.

The court proceedings were the outcome of an eighteen-month police investigation and referred to the period 1973–86 when Frank Beck worked for Leicestershire Social Services as an officer-in-charge of three children's homes. During much of this time he was regarded by the then management of Leicestershire Social Services as highly successful in dealing with difficult young people, using his own technique of 'regression therapy'. Some colleagues and former residents gave evidence in his defence. His local influence extended beyond the homes he ran: he chaired a departmental practice working party and, for a time, was a Liberal district councillor.

At the end of the trial, the Secretary of State ordered a national inquiry, to be held in private. He also instructed Leicestershire to hold a further inquiry, the county having already received a report from the former Deputy Director of Nottinghamshire Social Services, Barry Newell. The young people who suffered at Frank Beck's hands are expected to receive compensation from Leicestershire.

Although the trial of Frank Beck opened on 17 September 1991, reports did not appear in the news media until 27 September, when four national newspapers and the Press Association successfully challenged an order of the trial judge banning publicity about the case and about his own order. Some of the witnesses, although now in their twenties or thirties, were allowed to give evidence screened from the defendants.

The comparison of press coverage of the trial focuses particularly on the news treatment on the first day it was reported and on the outcome, with a more general review of the pattern of coverage during the proceedings. Five national daily papers are included, together with the *Leicester Mercury*, the local evening paper.

The Frank Beck trial opened less than four months after the publication of the Levy/Kahan report on pin-down. One might assume that this would have provided a ready-made framework for national press coverage in terms of ineptitude – or worse – in local government, professional influence built on bogus expertise, breach of trust, and the abuse of power (although it should be emphasized that there was never any suggestion that anyone involved in imposing pin-down was guilty of sexual offences). In the event, however, the treatment of the Frank Beck case was relatively low-key, which is, at first glance, the more surprising given the combination of human drama and sexual titillation available from the court case.

Of the national dailies sampled, *The Independent* came closest to giving the case the kind of play one would expect from its detailed coverage of the issues raised by pin-down and similar problems in residential child care. A prominent item on p. 1 focused on both the specifics of the appeal over the ban on publicity and its wider significance as a legal precedent. The case itself was given the top half of p. 3. There are three items with descriptive headlines, together with four photographs, of the defendants and of one of the homes. As with the pin-down affair, the more emotional aspects of the case are unusually foregrounded for a broadsheet. Although the longest item provides a summary of the case so far, two others provide sensational details: one about allegations concerning a local Labour MP, the other repeating some of the instances given in evidence. Both the detail and the language are far more explicit than anything that appeared in the mass tabloids or the local paper.

As the trial progressed, *The Independent* reported it on eleven further occasions. The items were relatively brief (about 15 column cm) but usually on p. 2 or 3, an indication of high-priority domestic news. Towards the end of October, the trial again became major news as Frank Beck gave evidence and allegations about the Labour MP were expanded. The four stories between 31 October and 12 November all included this feature of the case in the headline. There were no further reports until the verdict and sentence, which *The Independent* (30 November 1991) made its p. 1 lead: 'Head of children's homes jailed for life, five times', with the strapline 'Inquiries ordered into Britain's biggest sex abuse scandal "involving 200 victims"'. The text is in straight hard news format and is surprisingly brief, at 31 column cm. The accompanying picture of Beck leaving court is half as big again. There is no continuation inside the paper, no background, and no leader comment.

The pattern of *Daily Telegraph* coverage of the Frank Beck trial was very similar to that of *The Independent*. The response to the lifting of reporting restrictions was a summary of events so far, taking up nearly the whole of p. 3. '"13–year reign of terror" at children's homes' (*Daily Telegraph* 27 September 1991) and consisted of a bylined general account, parts of the evidence from four witnesses (only the one woman was not named), and a side column about the Labour MP. A large picture of Beck, framed by smaller shots of his co-accused and the three homes, completed the elaborate presentation.

The *Telegraph* reported the case on a further ten occasions during its progress, usually on p. 3 with the same byline. As with other papers, after the first couple of days, the trial became newsworthy only when Frank Beck gave evidence, the claims about the MP were raised again, and sentencing began. The end of the proceedings was reported in a flat descriptive item at the foot of p. 1 and a four-item assemblage filling the top half of p. 7, illustrated with pictures of Beck and the MP. The main story centres on administrative errors: 'Ex-social services chief provided two references for Beck' (*Daily Telegraph* 30 November 1991) and is an abbreviated account of some the issues discussed at length in the *Leicester Mercury* (see below). A 'profile' of Frank Beck and a history of the police investigation are also provided. The *Telegraph* made no editorial comment on the case.

On 27 September 1991, the *Daily Mail* placed its first report of the Frank Beck trial as the main item on p. 5: 'Sad children who were "warped by 13 years of abuse"' (a quotation from the prosecuting counsel), illustrated with a large picture of Beck. A white-on-black strapline added 'SOCIAL WORKER PUT TEENAGERS IN NAPPIES, COURT TOLD'. The text is, necessarily, a flat account of the proceedings by 'Daily Mail Reporter'. Only in the last paragraph is the lifting of the reporting ban mentioned, despite the obvious link with the Rochdale events. The *Mail* only mentioned the case four times as it developed; three of the stories related to the allegations about the MP, appearing on pp. 1, 2 and 5. On 27 November an illustrated report on p. 5 dealt with the conviction of Frank Beck's co-defendants.

The conclusion of the case occupied two-thirds of p. 2. The headline 'Blunders over Beck' (*Daily Mail* 30 November 1991) groups two stories and a picture of Beck. The longer, bylined, account opens with news of the government inquiries, moves on to some of the more startling revelations in the Newell inquiry report and mentions the NSPCC helpline being set up for 'victims of the Beck affair'. Only very brief details of the case are included. The shorter story refers to the Labour MP's forthcoming Commons statement. There is no further background beyond that available through official sources and no editorial comment.

The *Daily Mirror* and the *Sun* framed the case in remarkably similar fashion. On the first day that they could report it, both papers pegged the story to the allegations about the MP. The *Mirror* confined itself to a brief (11 column cm of text) description on p. 7, with a picture of the MP, while the *Sun* based 47 column cm on p. 11 on the evidence, headed '"CHILD SEX CASE MAN ROWED WITH BOY OVER LABOUR MP"', illustrated with the same picture. Thereafter the *Daily Mirror* mentioned the trial in progress on a further five occasions and the *Sun* four times, all of them triggered by fresh allegations about the link between a resident and the MP. Both papers made it a p. 1 item on one occasion. Otherwise it was relegated to pp. 4, 5, 7 and 15. On 9 November both mass tabloids made this subsidiary aspect of the trial the subject of large illustrated features.

The sentencing of Frank Beck was covered by the *Daily Mirror* in a dramatic presentation on p. 9 'LIFE ... FIVE TIMES' (in white-on-black); 'Sex brute caged for torment of kids in care' (*Daily Mirror* 30 November 1991), illustrated with a large picture of Beck. The main bylined story starts 'Evil Frank Beck was given five life sentences last night' and goes on to summarize the trial, its outcome and the launch of the official inquiries. A side column refers to the Labour MP dimension, with separate pictures of him and the young man concerned, and a third report highlights seven points from the internal inquiry report, under the heading 'SECRET OF BOSSES' FRANTIC COVER-UP'. There is no editorial comment.

Like the *Mirror*, the *Sun* combined an eye-catching presentation with a restrained text. Page 7 is dominated by a montage of a photo of Beck and the headline (in white-on-grey) 'Why was this man allowed to prey on young kiddies for 13 YEARS?' (*Sun* 30 November 1991). A smaller picture of one of the homes stands above a short account of the supposed 'regression therapy'. A second subsidiary report refers to the responses of the Secretary of State and of Leicestershire, quoting councillors and officers on likely compensation and changes that have been made. The main text is in hard news style, although larded with terms like 'damning', 'cover-up' and 'amazingly', combining details of the case with some of the findings of the internal inquiry report. The tone, though, is very low-key given the wealth of material on 'bungling bureaucrats' provided by the Newell report.

Although three journalists are credited with the copy, as in the other papers all the material could have come from routine court reports, the Newell report, news releases from the Secretary of State and from the Labour MP, and reports of the Leicestershire County Council press conference at the close of the trial. This impression of a lack of 'investigative work' is reinforced by mistakes about the name and former post of the internal 'scandal investigator' (*Sun* 30 November 1991) in both the *Sun* and the *Daily Mail*. Like other national dailies, the *Sun* made no editorial comment on the case.

The lack of detail in the national daily coverage of the Frank Beck trial is in marked contrast, not unexpectedly, with that provided by the *Leicester Mercury*. When reporting restrictions were lifted, the paper allocated nearly all of p. 1 and all the news space on four full pages to the proceedings so far, including long verbatim passages from (unnamed) witnesses. All the defendants, the judge and the homes were illustrated, and the significance of the issue further marked by giving it a logo of Justice with her sword and scales over the caption 'CHILDREN'S HOMES SEX ABUSE TRIAL'. (This was later changed to 'BECK CASE' over his picture.)

As the trial continued, the *Leicester Mercury* reported it almost every day. After the first three days of reporting, the coverage was on inside pages, but usually as the lead on the page, with the logo and often illustrated with photographs of the accused or one of the homes involved. At the end of October/beginning of November the case reappeared on p. 1 when Frank Beck gave evidence and was also front page news when the allegations about the local Labour MP were repeated in evidence. During most of the rest of November, when there was no mention in the national dailies, the *Leicester Mercury* frequently took up half a page or more with detailed accounts of the trial.

The final outcome of the case was the subject of a special edition of the local evening paper: 'TODAY WE PUBLISH THE SECRET REPORT ON THE BECK YEARS OF EVIL; Four pages of utterly compelling reading' – in a pull-out supplement (*Leicester Mercury* 30 November 1991). There were also four pages of news reports, the whole of pp. 1, 3, 4 and 5. Page 1 reproduced the comments of the judge in his summing-up and set out the charges and verdicts in detail. Page 3 covered similar details of the sentencing of Beck's co-defendants, above news of the Secretary of State's announcement of two inquiries. The lead on p. 4 is 'Abuse appalling says care chief at conference'. The conference itself is pictured, together with the director of social services, the county secretary, and representatives of all three county council political parties, who had attended the press conference. The main voice in the story is the director's, expressing revulsion and regret, and explaining what changes had been made to ensure no similar events could recur. Shorter articles cover other issues of high salience locally: details of the location and history of the four children's homes mentioned during the trial, and the likely cost to the council's insurers of compensating 'victims of Beck's reign of terror'.

Another very local aspect of the case occupies most of p. 5: the possibility that the inquest might be reopened on a boy who committed suicide, having run away from a home in Beck's charge. Several times more space is devoted to this by the *Leicester Mercury* than to another item on the page stating that police action was not to be taken against the Labour MP caught up in the case because of allegations by a defence witness.

The pull-out supplement is labelled 'Special Investigation' and provides a wealth of background detail and photographs: an interview with Beck while he was on remand; an 'exclusive interview' with the director of social services; a psychiatrist's explanation of the provenance of 'regression therapy'; a chronology; details of the scale of the police work preparing the case; lengthy extracts from the Newell report, including the contents of some of the letters on Frank Beck's personnel file, relating to controversial incidents – for example, a job reference that did not mention that he had been suspended before he had resigned; and a history of a fourth man who would have stood trial had he not left the UK and subsequently committed suicide.

On 30 November the *Leicester Mercury* devoted its leader column to 'Frank Beck: robber of childhood'. The editorial is written in the 'we' form as the voice of the community: 'It saddens and distresses and leaves us feeling empty that these words are being written about what happened in our county between 1973 and 1986'. It asks how 'senior County Council staff' could have known about complaints and done nothing, but then seems to widen blame out to everyone: 'Why did someone, anyone, not speak up and go on speaking and shouting up until those who would not hear took notice? Their silence has besmirched the name of Leicestershire.' The writer then looks forward to the inquiry, endorses the horror expressed by the director of social services, and assures county councillors that there will be 'no objection from the people' to funding any improvements that are needed.

INTERPRETING THE NEWS TREATMENT

Comparing the contours of the three cases, there would seem to be obvious parallels between the pin-down affair in Staffordshire and the failure to discover and terminate Frank Beck's exploitation of his positions in Leicestershire. Yet, as we have seen from the case studies, the similarities in intensity and tone of coverage in the national daily press are between the Rochdale events and pin-down. The clear implication is that it is less the events themselves than editorial priorities, news values and routines that have determined the press response.

What, then, are the common features of the Rochdale and pin-down scenarios? The first is the availability of a clear interpretative framework. This suggested itself immediately in the case of Rochdale: in their different ways the national papers treated it as a kind of 'hyper-Cleveland'. Commentators on the early press coverage of Cleveland (for example Nava 1988; Parton 1991) have demonstrated how, faced with disputes and unexpected alliances between normally credible and predictable sources, like doctors, police, and local politicians, the press reacted with an unusually open format of coverage. As the events unfolded a simplifying grid was gradually developed, imposed, and reinforced. For the tabloids, this was achieved by supporting the 'common sense' of local (male) politicians and the parents, and discrediting the (female) doctors and senior social workers. For the broadsheets the frame was well-founded expertise taken too far under the pressure of intense local controversy. The Butler Sloss report (Cm 412 1988) was then construed by the press as a final confirmation. All complexity (and subsequent developments, for which see Parton (1991)) were dissolved into an assumption that the social workers had panicked and been wrong.

By the time of Rochdale, 'satanic' abuse had already entered national debate. Authoritative voices like the Nottinghamshire police had, or could be understood to have, said that it did not exist. (The *Daily Mail* using the *Independent on Sunday* as authority was an intriguing spectacle.) Joining this to the conventions developed about the meaning of Cleveland produced a template of scepticism, if not outright rejection. In the case of the tabloids, any official criticism of the policies or practices of social services, whether from the police or the SSI, was simplified into condemnation. Actual condemnation uttered by a High Court judge was seized on as complete vindication of their own incredulity – even for the *Guardian*.

It is very striking that it took a long time for pin-down to pass the threshold of national press attention. Local political conflict and local media coverage had themselves triggered the television documentary. While even television documentaries are not 'blue sky research', there are the resources to assemble and present a much more complex scenario than is usual for everyday press investigations. Stakes like that of the *Financial Times* in the Maxwell affair are very exceptional. To an extent such television has traded on finding and naming new 'problems': an existing paradigm is not always required. Despite the television programme, for most of the national press, pin-down was not 'news' until the Levy/Kahan report transformed a provincial political wrangle into an easily grasped issue with national implications. Other happenings, like those at Ty Mawr, suddenly ceased to be haphazard, but part of a recognizable phenomenon. This is the 'sensitization' process identified in Cohen's (1973) account of the moral panic.

For once the tabloids and the broadsheets had common terrain: pin-down was simultaneously a problem of policy and politics, and also a heart-rending story of suffering children.

Over both Rochdale and pin-down the search for meaning by the national press was considerably helped by individuals and groups offering themselves as interpreters of events and spokespersons of aggrieved parties. Childwatch, PAIN and the Family Rights Group were all used as sources over the Rochdale events, their low status as small pressure groups presumably compensated for by the newspapers' predisposition towards the parents' case. Solicitors for the Rochdale families were also willing to talk to the media. And, as the *Guardian* huffily observed, some person or group involved in Rochdale was sophisticated enough about news media functioning to try to predetermine the media's 'reading' of the SSI report.

In Staffordshire there was no group, but a long and unpopular struggle by a local solicitor and a small number of local politicians. Once the issue was redefined as real by the authority of a QC and a child care expert, however, these were sources for the press to turn to – and some of the young people were willing to be identified and speak on their own behalf, as were some parents in Rochdale.

This, in turn, provided another key ingredient of news treatment: human interest and personalization. Resources were devoted to gathering and presenting this background colour by all the newspapers: features on the Rochdale estate concerned in the *Guardian* and the *Daily Telegraph*; interviews with subjects of pin-down in both *The Independent* and the *Daily Mirror*. For *The Independent* and the *Guardian* this enabled a twin-track approach. Many of their readers would be directly concerned with the professional dimensions of the affair, whether to do with the law, social work, or the administration of local government. They would have both professional and personal interest in the complexities of children's and parents' rights. But even broadsheet readers respond to family drama and children's pain; their visceral appeal serves to leaven otherwise abstract accounts.

Tabloids of the right and the left, as we have seen from earlier chapters, use individual experience and behaviour, not only to frame news coverage, but to explain the events and the world itself. The *Daily Mirror*'s continuing support for a socialist perspective, however diluted, produces the kind of ambiguities of interpretation not demonstrated by the *Daily Mail*. Thus on the same page the *Mirror* vilified Tony Latham for developing and administering pin-down but also argued powerfully that poor residential care is a collective response to a collectively generated problem for which we should all accept responsibility.

The *Daily Mail* also had to make difficult choices, to reject some attractive targets in order to strike at others. Too much detail on the full horrors of 'Socialist Staffordshire' (30 May 1991) would have obscured the blameworthiness of individuals.

Child protection work dominates both state social work and the voluntary sector. In turn, the fiercest debate about its practice pivots on the respective rights of parents and children. A further explanation of the isomorphism of news processing between Rochdale and pin-down was the apparent ease with which the national press could resolve this issue and invite the reader to support an apparently self-evident good. In Rochdale 'common sense', then the police, and finally the authority of the judiciary indicated that the parents had been wronged. Once the Levy/Kahan investigation had castigated pin-down as an illegal abuse of both individual and system power, papers of the left and the right, broadsheet and tabloid, could champion the whole class of young people concerned against individual social workers and local authority bureaucracy. For the broadsheets, and perhaps the *Daily Mirror*, children having civil rights is a thinkable thought. It was this, rather than a simple attack on state welfare, that drove the high volume of attention given to pin-down and related cases in *The Independent* and, conversely, inhibited the *Guardian* from an immediate assumption that there was no foundation to social services' concerns in Rochdale.

For the mid-market tabloids, especially the *Daily Mail*, parents are assumed to have inherently greater rights than children, enshrined in the property rights of the conventional patriarchal family – unless they forfeit them by being part of the deviant minority. The pin-down case, though, was appealingly simple. As parents hardly appeared in the action at all, the possibility that Staffordshire had been correct to take the young people into care, even if failing the management of that care, never needed to be considered. Even wrong-doing young people could be forgiven, on the 'mine enemy's enemy' principle.

'Something must be done' and 'we told you so' are important organizing themes of leader comment. Both Rochdale and pin-down offered a wealth of possibilities for editorial indignation: demands for the disciplining of staff, for changes in social work training; party political attacks; support for government guidance and legislation; even, in the *Daily Mirror*, calls for wholesale social change.

The local politics of the issue is another common feature of the Rochdale and pin-down sagas. Both cases were highly politicized, with a ruling Labour group, internal dissent and abundant public mutual accusation. For most of the tabloids this was satisfactory in itself; the *Daily Mirror* had to perform a more delicate balancing act, trying to hold the line between villains and victims, but keeping the welfare bureaucracy defined as doing a necessary and difficult job. In the broadsheets it fitted the presumed general interest of the readership in the political process; party-political blame merely adds fascination. However, as the case material on court cases involving a child's death shows, the way a newspaper responds to events is not simply a matter of reading off its politics. The treatment of Rochdale and pin-down also clearly underlines that newspaper agendas and values are set within a finely tuned appreciation of their market.

We have seen *The Independent*'s determinedly progressive stance over children's rights. Since it is the paper's unique selling proposition that it does not systematically support any party, the political quagmires in Rochdale and Staffordshire were not a problem. Is it assumed by extension that *The Independent*'s readers are closet individualists, more interested than they would admit in the private and experiential? This would certainly explain the volume of human interest that the paper provided, not just over pin-down and Rochdale but the Frank Beck trial as well.

It is a long-standing joke that leaders in the *Guardian* can sustain several opinions at once. Yet over Rochdale, after an initial struggle, the paper leapt to the parents' defence, ditching the concerns of its stereotype readership. One possible explanation of this apparent paradox is the newspaper's roots, as the *Manchester Guardian*, in the north-west. As a result, over Rochdale, it reacted more like a local paper than a liberal national broadsheet. The police rejection of the satanism allegations was not sufficient for the paper to abandon the intricacies of professional debate (especially since there was no love lost between the *Manchester Evening News* and the then Chief Constable), but, once given permission by a High Court judge, populism could be embraced.

The *Daily Telegraph* is well known as a Conservative paper. Nevertheless, its account of Rochdale (apart from a bit of ritualized old-bufferism in leader and headlines) worked away from simplification to complexity. Its reporting of pin-down was informative but low-key, treating it as a political issue with both local and national implications. The *Telegraph* is not the paper of the caring professions, as is obvious from the range of staff used to cover a social services issue. It is, rather, the paper of the knights of the shires, many of whom are politicians themselves. Conservative local authorities have social services departments too, so there would be little mileage in rubbishing the *idea* of social work. Besides, the *Telegraph* is inclined towards the one-nation Toryism which endorses collective provision, albeit motivated by paternalism rather than the eradication of inequality.

The mid-market tabloids are the papers of small proprietors and middle-level functionaries. For them the state is a parasite, thwarting their efforts to be self-sufficient with its labyrinthine restrictions and the tax demands made to support both itself and the indigent who will not struggle on their own behalf. Both the *Daily Express* and the *Daily Mail* make a virtue out of reaction: their tone is angry, particularly about what are presented as corrupting progressive ideas in education, criminal justice and the welfare state. 'Traditional' family values are constantly paraded, not only over parents' rights, but in a persistent, insidious ridiculing of women who step outside conventional gender patterns. (This alone might explain the unexpected gradual success of the previously struggling *Today* in this sector of the market.) Attacks on state social work are thus likely to resonate with *Mail* and *Express* readers on several levels.

The mass tabloids do not have a consistent campaign against state social work: like other complex aspects of the social and political system, it becomes tabloid news when it is transformed into a dramatic (preferably sexual or criminal) episode between identifiable persons. As we have seen, far from giving Judge Douglas Brown's scathing criticism of socialist welfare work the big treatment, the *Sun* barely registered it. The *Daily Mirror* is unpredictable as it tries to balance right-wing Labour sensibility with wholesome, folksy populism, and also compete with the more unrestrained style of the *Sun* for its share of a shrinking market.

Given this sketch of the market-driven concerns of the national newspapers, one would surely imagine that the mass tabloids, at least, would have been ready with pages of coverage at the end of the Frank Beck trial, as they were over Tyra Henry (see Chapter 2), the Colin Evans/Marie Payne case (see Chapter 5) and many other sensational sex-crime trials (Soothill and Walby 1991). But they did not react in this way, despite ample time, and a ready-made paradigm, based on pin-down as 'things go badly wrong in state residential care', offering itself. Some components of an explanation are offered below, but I continue to find this case profoundly puzzling.

The mundane mechanics of the newsgathering process suggests a partial explanation. The Frank Beck trial lacked some of the concrete components for major news treatment, and limited the openings for editorial postures.

Those who had been violated by Frank Beck appeared to have no groups or individuals speaking specifically for them, offering a construction of events to the press. Indeed it was the very isolation and powerlessness of Frank Beck's victims that had enabled him to exploit them for so long. In the end it was a chance remark to the social services department, three years after Frank Beck had left Leicestershire, that triggered the last and effective police investigation. There had been no response to those young people and staff who had protested during his reign.

The prosecution witnesses in the Beck case had not only been traumatized but also felt shamed. Some newspapers named witnesses when reporting the trial; others did not. Neither they nor their relatives could easily be used for conventional 'colour' stories. Yet this cannot be the whole explanation. Soothill and Walby (1991: 60) describe the avalanche of coverage that followed the conviction of a serial rapist. Even though his trial only lasted one day, and the identities of those he raped (although not those he sexually assaulted) were legally protected, the *Sun* 'had seven pages (including a special four-page pull-out)'.

The injunction banning publicity at the start of the Frank Beck trial was modified, not wholly lifted. It is not clear whether background stories and editorializing were inhibited by the reporting restrictions – but the *Leicester Mercury* was able to print a leader. One of the staff involved in reporting the case does not recall any specific restraints lasting beyond the trial itself.

Presumably trying to develop the angle of the case involving the Labour MP would have risked a libel action because of his consistent denial that there was any truth in the claims of the defence witness.

Perhaps we should move from the mechanics of news to its ideological assumptions. Did Frank Beck's victims, being young people in care, lack both sentimental appeal and citizenship claims, especially for the tabloids? This further angle still does not provide a complete answer: even the *Daily Mail* showed some interest in the civil rights of the young people subjected to pin-down.

The political dimensions of the case were certainly attenuated by the limited opportunities to demand action, whether a tabloid-style search for blameworthy individuals, or the broadsheets' standard demand for policy review. Frank Beck was found guilty and received a very heavy sentence. The government had acted through the Secretary of State's call for two further inquiries. Leicestershire County Council had accepted full responsibility and taken action through an internal investigation; many of the senior social services managers who had failed to stop Beck had been replaced. The local politics of the affair are obviously crucial, but remained inward-turned. It is not possible from reading newspaper reports to detect which was the majority party in the county. There must have been bitter recriminations but they are not apparent. The *Leicester Mercury*'s account of the post-trial press conference shows a pointed demonstration of all-party solidarity. Is this one of the key differences from the pin-down affair?

Surely, though, even if some of the components were not there for tabloid investigative journalism, the Newell report would have been of interest to the broadsheets as policy/politics, and to both mid- and mass-market tabloids as a gross example of 'bureaucratic bungling'? There seems to have been no attempt to keep it as an internal document: long passages appeared in the *Leicester Mercury*. Nor was social services management refusing to discuss the case. The Newell report contained blunt criticisms – it could hardly be written off as a whitewash. Yet only the *Daily Telegraph* gave this aspect of the case prominent treatment. Or do the national broadsheets and the *Daily Mail* simply not regard an internal inquiry by a provincial fellow professional as an authoritative source?

Can possible legal restraints, the imperatives of the news production process, and lack of overt political feuding by themselves explain the curiously muted response of the national press to Frank Beck? (And of social work's own press, which has given the case much less space than its importance would seem to warrant.)

Here, surely, was a man whose behaviour precisely fitted the category of 'monster' used, particularly in the tabloid press, to explain and contain sex crime as a matter of individual psychopathology (Soothill and Walby 1991)? And, moreover, he was a qualified social worker. The mid- and mass-market Tory tabloids are usually pleased to report accusations of wrong-doing against anyone remotely connected with the caring business. For example, the p. 1 lead of the *London Standard* (now the *Evening Standard*) on 25 June 1986 read 'IS STRANGLER A SOCIAL WORKER?', a reference to a line of police thinking on a series of murders. Post-office clerk and civil servant were also being canvassed.

Did Frank Beck confound the press by bursting out of the monster paradigm? Extravagant language ('monster' itself, 'evil', 'animal'), used in the tabloid descriptions of men like Andrew Neil, David Salt and Colin Evans, obscures the underlying assumption that the existence of such deviants is 'normal'. By a paradox their behaviour, although extreme, is banal and containable. Monsters are axiomatically few in number. All about sex, the trial was ironically unmanageable for the tabloids, which are saturated with sex but fundamentally puritan in their treatment of it. This man with a voracious and bisexual appetite could not be neatly categorized. He is an ex-Marine, white and educated, has been married, has been successful and respected. He looks worryingly unlike an alien. Yet he committed appalling crimes over a long period, mostly against young men but also a young woman. For the tabloids, in short, he undermines the comforting solidity of the normality/deviance, us/them divide.

For the broadsheets it could be argued that Frank Beck was also uncontainable, but in a different way. It is one thing to condemn breach of trust when a building society manager does a bunk with a helping of the branch deposits. It is another to contemplate the implications of a man working for thirteen years as a respected professional colleague and local politician while committing dreadful offences, not in another private and secret domain, but in the workplace, some of them against fellow employees. The obvious question is, as in Cleveland: how many more? Whereas this is a harmless rhetorical device for the protagonists in an everyday moral panic, in the Frank Beck case an answer could challenge the integrity of the social fabric.

Chapter 4

Elderly people – the invisible clients

From their trade journals and everyday discourse, it is evident that social workers' fear of hostile news media coverage is powerful and pervasive. As we have seen from earlier chapters, the anxiety generated by the most highly publicized trials following the death of a child has produced an inclusive mythology. Crucial – and potentially reassuring – questions about which media, in what circumstances, about what clients, of which agencies, are not thought through. It is already clear (and will become more so when the probation service and voluntary agencies are considered in later chapters) that, where there has been aggressive news treatment, it has focused on local authority social services. Does this mean that all national daily papers have an automatic predisposition to be at least critical (in the case of the centre left press and the broadsheets) or condemnatory (in the case of the Tory tabloid press) of everything that social services does, simply because it *is* social services? If so, we should expect that, when mistakes are made or controversial policies pursued in respect of client groups other than children, then the national press would use similar templates of coverage.

Of the many responsibilities of local authority social services, work with elderly people is the most significant competitor of child protection in terms of resources, especially as the major changes involved in community care policies are installed. With this in mind, I tried to find instances where social services could be seen as having failed in work with elderly people, or were being campaigned against, to compare the extent and style of press treatment. This of course raised in a more acute form the same methodological problem as the case studies of child protection work: how does one know of episodes which are not covered by the news media? Inevitably, then, the three examples of national news coverage considered below had received some media attention. The insight they provide comes from its scope, compared with arguably similar circumstances involving children.

TALK OF THE DEVIL IN HAMMERSMITH AND FULHAM

On 8 June 1992 the *Guardian* reported, under the headline 'Social workers failed woman who saw devil', that the Local Government Ombudsman had found 'the London borough of Hammersmith and Fulham guilty of maladministration causing injustice'. The article, on an inside news page and bylined 'Social Services Correspondent', provided considerable detail (27 column cm) about the case. The landlord, and later the bank manager, of an elderly local resident had contacted social services to report that she was becoming confused and aggressive, and not caring for herself. At the initial contact a recently qualified locum social worker had 'failed to complete a referral form for further action'. After five months, the landlord was troubled enough to contact his MP. The following month the situation had deteriorated to the extent that social services, with the police and a psychiatrist, had to break into the woman's flat and take her to hospital. As a result, Hammersmith and Fulham conducted an investigation and made policy changes. Apart from the concern expressed that the elderly woman was not offered help, the Ombudsman's report criticized the borough for its '"haphazard"' case review procedures and for causing worry and inconvenience to the woman's landlord, housing manager and fellow tenants.

This episode would seem to have many features to attract national press coverage. Salience for the broadsheets was demonstrated by the *Guardian*, as the case raised policy and professional issues, combined with colourful human interest details. According to its report, these included the woman thinking that one of the social workers was 'the daughter of Dracula', which is ready-made for a mass tabloid headline. And of course this was bureaucratic bungling, officially recognized, which might have appealed to the mid-market dailies. The events had also taken place in London, which tends to signify with the national press, and would make for easy follow-up. Nevertheless, on 8 and 9 June 1992, the case was not reported by any of the other papers sampled: the *Daily Telegraph*, the *Daily Mail*, the *Sun* or the *Daily Mirror*.

Among possible reasons for the lack of press response to the Ombudsman's report might be the contemporary furore about Andrew Morton's biography of the Princess of Wales, and that the Ombudsman's report did not name any of the parties in the case, making further investigation more difficult for journalists. This latter point manifestly does not apply to elderly people actively seeking publicity for their campaign against social services' actions.

BATTLING FOR RIGHTS IN DEVON AND DURHAM

Community Care of 9 July 1992 reported that in an 'important test case' about to end in the High Court, 'five elderly women, three from Devon and two from Durham, challenged decisions by their county councils to close residential care homes, claiming no effort had been made to consult them'. The residents, aged between 82 and 92 years, were seeking judicial review. In the event, the case was dismissed, 'leaving no doubt that local authorities have the legal right to close their residential homes without consultation', otherwise '"administrative chaos"' would result (*Community Care* 16 July 1992). According to the judge, not only are local authorities democratically elected, but residents could also complain to the Secretary of State for Health. As the *Community Care* article emphasizes, however, an important moral issue was raised. Current legislation requires children to be consulted before parallel decisions are taken about the future of their residential care homes. According to the chair of the ADSS elderly persons' committee, consulting elderly people should also become standard practice.

Here, again, would seem to be the components of a good story. Some of the residents demonstrated outside the High Court with placards about being 'evicted': pictures are provided in *Community Care*. Elderly pickets have novelty value, surely? (Clichés about 'battling grannies' crowd to mind.) It is not simply a tabloid exaggeration to say that such home closures can have life-or-death implications for residents, whose health may be seriously affected by such disruption – a point made to *Community Care* by the voluntary agency for elderly people, Counsel and Care. If it is high on a newspaper's editorial agenda, local government can easily be portrayed as inhumane and doctrinaire in this situation. National policy matters were also at stake, as the closures resulted from the redirection of funds towards other aspects of community care. That there can be plenty of mileage and several angles to such scenarios is evident from the intense local press coverage of a similar row in Nottinghamshire, recounted below. Despite this, my scrutiny of the *Guardian*, the *Daily Telegraph*, the *Daily Mail*, the *Sun* and the *Daily Mirror* for the period 8 to 16 July 1992 failed to locate any mention of the Devon/Durham court case, the campaign, or its human consequences, on their news pages.

Perhaps, drawing a parallel with the deaths of children known to the local authority, what is needed for press attention is an apparent mistake, with implied blame, and very unpleasant consequences.

DEATH IN THE WIRRAL

The *Daily Telegraph* of 9 July 1991 reported, in a bylined item on p. 5, that a resident in sheltered housing had been dead for six weeks before being discovered. Care for residents was provided by the staff of an adjacent social services elderly persons' home, linked by a call system. The events were clearly serious in the eyes of the local authority. According to the Director of Wirral Borough Council Social Services in the *Telegraph* report, "'We are extremely concerned at what has happened and I have instituted a full inquiry into the sad death of this old lady.'" (The inquiry subsequently found no individual to be responsible, but procedures were improved.)

Instances where people have lain dead and undiscovered are often reported in the press, both tabloid and broadsheet, because of the drama and identification: it could be you or a relative, or you could be the worried neighbour. For this to happen in sheltered housing makes blaming social services easy. As we have seen, the mid-market tabloids are not usually inhibited by lack of detailed knowledge from going into the attack. This case made national television news, but apart from the *Daily Telegraph* report described above, I could find no reference to it in the *Guardian*, the *Daily Mail*, the *Sun* or the *Daily Mirror* for 9 or 10 July 1992.

Evidently social services work with elderly people, even when it is dramatic 'bad news' or heart-tugging human interest, does not often pass the threshold of significance for the national dailies, because of their interwoven market niche, editorial policies and news values. Identical circumstances can, however, be very big news indeed for local media. The 1990–1 saga of Nottinghamshire County Council's elderly persons' homes was the subject of the local paper's equivalent of tabloid 'monstering'.

'SAVE OUR HOMES': THE UNFOLDING NEWS

On 1 November 1990 the front page lead of the Nottingham *Evening Post* (hereafter *EP*) was 'DON'T RUIN OUR LIVES', with the strapline a 'Tearful plea from Beattie, 99', who also asked (in an inset headline) "'Why can't they leave us alone?'" A very large picture of her, wiping her eyes, dominated the page. At issue was a report, to go before the county's social services committee the following week, recommending closure of thirteen of the authority's elderly persons' homes. After the highly personalized opening paragraphs, the news treatment described the regret of the committee chair and explained events in terms of the costs of new central government-imposed standards.

The news was continued in a 'Special Report', credited to two named and pictured woman journalists. It fills p. 15, accompanied by four pictures of residents, with the headline 'Fears and tears at the old folk's homes; 350 pensioners face the shock of having to move; "It will be the death of me"' dominating a text organized almost entirely around personal cases. The proposed closures are also the subject of that day's editorial, which is magisterial: 'Compromise to cut the heartbreak'. The paper congratulates itself for not '"going for the jugular"' of the social services chair. Instead, having acknowledged the difficult position of the authority and the good intentions behind the government legislation, it pleads with those concerned to 'put politics aside and get together to explore every conceivable alternative to putting the old folk through such misery'. After all, 'Nottinghamshire is not an irresponsible, rabid-Left local authority'.

This self-consciously balanced stance was underlined the following day (2 November 1990) when the (pictured) chair of social services was given most of an inside page to explain 'My agony over closed homes'. She lists legislation, a limited budget, empty places in some homes, and principled opposition to privatization as reasons for her '"sleepless nights"' and 'months of agony' over the '"heartbreaking"' decision. A small amount of space is given to a local Conservative group reaction and a comment from Labour-controlled neighbouring Derbyshire.

The committee decision to go ahead with most of the closure programme appeared on p. 1 as 'Heartbreak for Lily' (*EP* 8 November 1990). The detail appeared on p. 5, now relegated to 'Post Reporter', and headed 'Old folk defy council', with a picture of protesting staff and residents. A number of voices are quoted: residents, staff, the unions, the opposition Conservative group and dissident Labour councillors, but the official explanations are given plenty of space in standard for-and-against style. The leader is again devoted to the controversy and claims to be 'objective and politically impartial', chiding the elected members for not taking the editorial advice of the previous week. But, says the writer, while the paper is impartial, it is not neutral about the welfare of the 'old people' who may 'have to endure the heartbreak of being split up from the friends who are their "family" and moved from the homes in which they feel safe, familiar and secure'. Despite its promised neutrality, the leader introduces some very political questions about the priorities within the overall budget, the selling of homes, and policies elsewhere. 'Balance' is reimposed by calling on the government to make Nottinghamshire a special case.

By 12 November, the terms of the dispute were shifting: 'Public joins homes fight' featured prominently on the front page, with a continuation inside. Although still in hard news style, the pro-closure case was limited to one paragraph; the rest reported the 'battle plan' by the staff, residents, relatives, and local sitting and prospective MPs. The 'public's' contribution seemed to be limited to signing petitions.

Suddenly, on 20 November, the intensity of coverage was stepped up. It had become a campaign, complete with logo: 'Save Our Homes' as the caption to a cropped version of the day one picture of Beattie wiping her eyes. 'WE STRIKE IF HOMES CLOSE' was the very large p. 1 lead. Inside, a complete page is given to local Conservative councillors maintaining that 'Cash could have been found'. The editorial is headed 'Council must find an alternative' and opens with the claim that, should the strike take place, 'public support for such action would surely be 100 per cent. And when did that last happen with industrial action?' In highly emotive terms, the leader goes on to characterize the residents 'who ask no more than to be left alone in their own homes' as caught between the county council and the government. The paper not only congratulates the unions for 'not using the situation to indulge in government-bashing' but identifies itself with them: 'like the *Post* the unions can see both political sides to this story . . . It's a welcome illustration of the constructive and sensible behaviour which is becoming the hallmark of modern trades unionism.' Can this be the same Nottingham *Evening Post* that was involved in a bitter dispute with its journalists during the imposition of new technology in the mid-1970s and was, for several years, the subject of a national trade union and Labour Party boycott?

The *Post* campaign report' of 27 November was headed 'HAVE A HEART FOR OLD FOLK' and asserted 'pressure on Labour county councillors to reverse their decision is intensifying'. 'Post campaign; D-Day December 20' had now been added to the logo, should anyone have failed to notice the military build-up. Presumably because it was now a 'campaign', hard news style had been abandoned in favour of exhortations to Labour councillors to break ranks, and to readers to write in. The director of social services is described as 'claiming', words like 'ludicrously' are included, and the paper's scepticism of the majority party's position is conveyed by distancing inverted commas: 'They have set up a "working party"'; 'The Tories, the *Post*, the residents have until December 20 to reach the consciences of just seven Labour councillors'. Residents are, it seems, not centre-stage any more. (Also on 27 November, two news items reported the activities of various local politicians and the story of an individual resident, 'still reeling from the shock'.)

The emotional pressure was increased still further on 28 November with a front page account of a demonstration outside County Hall, together with 'PLEASE LET US STAY TOGETHER' above a very large picture of two women residents and their 'BEST PALS PLEA TO COUNCIL' in five paragraphs above the campaign logo. On p. 1 two articles juxtapose the picture and point of view of one of the 'brave-faced' residents who has been actively campaigning – '"I would rather die than leave here. I've had a hard enough life as it is. The staff here are like my daughters, the residents are like my sisters and brothers"' – and the chair of social services, who is given considerable space to rehearse the reasons for 'My regret but axe has to fall'.

The chair of social services was described on 29 November as 'FACE TO FACE WITH ANGER' by agreeing to attend a village meeting with the director. Most of the text is given to a local councillor organizing the protest. A side column, below the inset logo, provides another personal reaction from a named resident.

Proposed industrial action by NALGO and NUPE was the p. 1 lead on 30 November 1990. The trade unions are quoted sympathetically and the action portrayed as simultaneously highly disruptive and not intended to cause real suffering. Another 'campaign' article inside gives extensive coverage to the possible consequences of the homes closure on a named and pictured couple. The leader column also advocates their case: 'In the context of their age, they are "newlyweds" – having been married just 18 years.' Later in the editorial, after support for the industrial action, a new criticism of the county council is introduced: that no other authority is closing as many homes. It concludes by again declaring the paper's apolitical stance and proudly pleading guilty to being 'simplistic and emotional'.

On 5 December the paper's coverage lived up to this declaration: 'THEY CRIED LIKE BABIES; But these were tears of joy'. The cause was the decision of the county council Labour group to give three (of the thirteen) homes a 'definite reprieve' and three more a '"stay of execution"'. About two-thirds of the very lengthy article was given to the reactions of residents, staff and unions, with the remainder containing explanations from local politicians of how the money was to be found. The day's editorial describes the 'U-turn' as being to the 'eternal credit' of the social services chair, after 'one of the biggest public campaigns ever seen in the county'. The following day (6 December) an inside page article, headed 'WE FIGHT ON VOW OLD FOLK' and illustrated with two pictures of groups of residents, combined further individual testimonies with political claim and counter-claim.

'D-Day 20 December' marked the crucial meeting of the full council, so the issue was reintroduced as news on 17 December by a brief item about a NUPE/county council meeting. It reads oddly, in terms of presentational conventions, as the headline plus logo occupy more column space than the text. On 18 December another pot-boiler article, gathering together a number of minor developments, appeared on p. 5. Again on 20 December a similar piece summarized events so far and quoted opposition voices.

When the debate and vote came, the Labour majority on the county council held, so: 'Save the homes bid fails; But Tories and old folk vow to fight on' (*EP* 21 December 1990). The high-profile news treatment started with the second lead on p. 1, took up much of p. 3 and was supported by an editorial comment which signalled the weight given to the issue by beginning on p. 1. The main theme of the leader is a personal attack on the chair of social services. She is accused in the opening sentence of having 'perfected the art of passing the buck . . . Throughout she has shifted all the blame and all the responsibility on to the government. And now she is blaming the *Evening Post*!' The writer stoutly reaffirms its 'apolitical stance': 'Right from the beginning our position has been the same. We have said all along that the only people who matter are the old folk in those homes.' The responsibility cannot be the government's, the writer argues, or the unions would have 'heaped all the blame on to their inherent Tory enemies'. The 'U-turn', previously praised as good sense, is transformed into evidence that there was no need to close the homes in the first place. Most of the reasons brought forward by the Labour group are now interpreted and presented as 'excuses'. Again the paper points out that it has not '"crucified"' the chair of social services although 'It is true that the *Post*'s Comment on the issue became more pungent as the story developed. That was not some populist reaction to public hostility over the closures.'

News coverage on 21 December consisted of three items. The first half of the front page hard news story pursues the 'fight on' theme. The financial and policy complexities of the issue are rolled up with the political dispute in the latter half, as the story continues on p. 3. On that page the first lead is '*Post* under fire on homes crisis', which describes part of the chair of social services' contribution to the council meeting. The opposition point of view is spelled out in another story, without the conventional balance of a Labour reply: 'LABOUR BROKE ITS PROMISES – TORIES'.

According to the standing orders of Nottinghamshire County Council, a further debate on the closure of the elderly person's homes could not be held for six months. In July 1991 the controversy reappeared as the p. 1 lead '"WE'LL SAVE OLD FOLK'S HOMES"' (*EP* 18 July 1991), reporting the possibility that 'A dozen Labour county councillors plan to support moves to keep the old people's homes open – against their leader's policy.' The lengthy hard news story quotes both political camps and sketches the previous history of the dispute. Despite the previous efforts of the paper, this account of the reopening of the issue is not accorded a bylined report and the logo is not used.

In the July vote sufficient Labour county councillors abstained or supported the Conservative motion to overturn the closure policy. This was greeted by the *Evening Post* (19 July 1991) with a dramatic p. 1 treatment. A very large head-and-shoulders picture of two residents raising their glasses in a toast overlaps the large (3 cm type) headline '"STAY PUT" OLD FOLK ARE TOLD', in white-on-grey. 'Rejoicing' residents feature in the first paragraph; 'The Labour leadership's first policy defeat in ten years came during a 20-hour meeting – the longest in the county council's history' was the second. A summary of events and positions follows, with more details of the debate on p. 5.

The inevitable leader comment is, however, equivocal rather than triumphalist. Instead of adopting the 'campaigning' style of the previous December, the inflection is the judicious 'balance' of the opening stages of the affair. 'The plight of those 350 elderly people was a cause this newspaper willingly championed. But in so doing, we recognised that the issues were not black and white ... We were reluctant to apportion blame.' The reprise of the imbroglio still focuses on the 'peace of mind' of the residents, but rehabilitates the chair of social services as having been in a difficult situation, and attributes good intentions to the precipitating government legislation. The paper characterizes its campaign as a moral stance, facilitated by empirical weaknesses in the closure policy, and further justified by the support of councillors, trade unions and 'scores of *Post* readers'. The closing section reads:

> Now, amid the political wreckage, Labour must start on the 'almost impossible' task of finding the £1 million needed to keep those homes open ... something must give – and that means it may not be just *political* futures at risk. The courage of those Labour rebels cannot be denied. Now they, and the county council must weigh up the cost.
>
> (*EP* 19 July 1991; emphasis in original)

'SAVE OUR HOMES': INTERPRETING THE NEWS TREATMENT

The most immediately interesting feature of the Nottingham *Evening Post*'s response to the elderly person's homes controversy is the move from detailed but neutral reporting to a strident campaign – and then back to a more low-key approach. To manage these changes of perspective, however, important aspects of the landscape had to remain stable and be rendered apparently simple.

If elderly persons' homes are to be defended, they must be at least adequate; in fact they were portrayed as perfect. From the coverage, it seems that all Nottinghamshire homes were completely without fault, and all staff not merely kind and skilled, but superb – even when active trade unionists. Not only domestic but family terminology is frequently used. There is an irony here, as 'putting your relative in a home' is not approved of in right-wing populist versions of the exemplary family. It is clear from the news stories that not only do some of the residents have living relatives, but some are primary kin and are playing a part in the campaign. They are rarely foregrounded or quoted, though.

The homogenization and idealization of the staff and the homes in the news accounts is, however, as nothing compared with that applied to the residents. Fowler's (1991) work on news language is helpful here, in particular his dissection of the way that hospital patients are constructed as passive, even in a news text that intends sympathetically to challenge the political and medical hierarchy on their behalf. Clearly one must be cautious about drawing parallels: it suited campaigning Nottinghamshire residents, staff and others to emphasize deservingness and dependency. The language of the *Evening Post* often goes beyond this. It is very sentimental (a feature also of the media framing of disabled people – see Cumberbatch and Negrine (1992)); it implies gratitude rather than the citizenship right of support; it constructs old age in terms of childhood – sometimes explicitly, as in 'THEY CRIED LIKE BABIES' (*EP* 5 December 1990). Elderly people, although often referred to thus in the text, are always 'old folk' in headlines, with the resultant 'old folk's homes'. Their names are rendered forename–surname at the first mention, but they are often referred to subsequently by forename only, which does not happen to the chair of social services, even when being attacked in highly personal terms. Such familiarity, as Fowler (1991) also points out, is applied at the extremes of social standing: children, servants, and the very famous indeed: Di; Gazza.

It would be unreasonable to criticize the *Evening Post* for citing the age of residents. This is routine when previously unknown people enter the public arena, and is salient to the issue. It is, though, very striking that age is usually the only attribute referred to (other than gender). Even the male residents are not credited with a previous occupation, for example, nor any current activities or interests. The few adjectives used about residents included: 'frail', 'sick', 'talkative', 'hardy and determined', 'brave-faced', 'twice-widowed', 'blind', 'worried', 'chatty'.

Again the newspaper can hardly be blamed for taking up the theme of the residents' wish – at least in the case of those satisfied enough to be willing to be identified – for stability and familiarity. This could have been presented in positive terms: some of the personal testimonies that feature so prominently in the news treatment point out that moving into the home had been a deliberate choice, which was now being undone. But the linguistic style of the news stories constantly stresses the 'done to', vulnerability, and passivity. Residents want to be 'left alone' and 'safe and secure'; they are 'cared for', 'victims', and 'taken for coffee'; they are 'dreading', 'worried', 'heartbroken', 'tearful', 'inconsolable', have 'fears'. Weeping became a recurrent symbol in pictures and headlines. Most of the pictures show residents inactive, with wheelchairs and Zimmer frames included in a number of instances. One of the few more assertive poses is, interestingly, of a man jabbing his finger to emphasize his point of view. Women usually gaze soulfully at the camera.

Conversely, other parties to the dispute were lexicalized as active to the point of extreme violence. The goodies had 'campaigns' and 'battle-plans' – even 'D-Day'. Allusions to these often included the residents of the homes, but not as first in the list of combatants. The baddies were going to 'axe', 'execute' or, hopefully, 'reprieve' the homes.

From the start this was treated as a human drama, saturated with stereotyped emotions. The issues were, as we shall further explore below, very simplified. Much of this simplification was achieved, as it is in the national tabloid press, by personalization. The campaign was fought by constant reference to the effects of closure on individuals; particular members of staff were also called in aid. On the 'other side', the immensely complex financial, policy and political issue was framed throughout as the individual responsibility of the chair of social services. Even the leader of the Labour group on the county council was not given much prominence, despite the crucial decisions being taken in full council. Nor was the chair of the finance committee mentioned more than briefly. The same semi-invisibility applied to social services professional staff. The director was the only named person identified with the department; he was alluded to five times, and then briefly and in a subsidiary role. This even extended to the one instance where he was quoted, saying on the last day of coverage that: 'discussions would begin today about how the money could be found to keep the homes open' (*EP* 19 July 1991).

This absence is of pivotal importance for the understanding of the press and social work. The homes were the responsibility of social services, the staff were social services employees and some of them probably social work qualified, the policy came from social services management as a result of government policy, and yet, during the whole saga, 'social work' or 'social workers' were hardly mentioned. 'Save Our Homes' was not social work news but local politics. Nevertheless, a closer look at the stance of the local paper in the political scenario has important implications for comprehending the actual and potential relationship between social services and local media.

The proposal to close elderly persons' homes was the precipitate of not one but a number of policies and political processes reacting together. The first to be quoted in the newspaper coverage as an explanation were the new government requirements for the buildings themselves, combined with falling occupancy as a result of community care developments. Privatization was also an issue from the start, in that it was not an option to be considered. As time went on, other factors entered the frame: central government restrictions on borrowing; central government limitations on spending, with consequent risks of penalties for over-spending; the amounts paid by DSS in support of residents in local authority sector, as opposed to private or voluntary agency, residential care; and competing demands on the social services budget. Yet, despite this being 'one of the biggest campaigns ever seen in the county' (*EP* 5 December 1990), it is very striking how small a proportion of the news space was given to setting out these issues for readers. Some of them, notably the financial formulae, are complex to the extent that professionals struggle over them. Others, like community care, are capable of translation into accessible lay terms. Privatization would also seem an obvious angle, particularly as it has been pursued by other local authorities and was advocated by the *Evening Post* itself.

Even if the policy background was complex, this cannot be an adequate explanation for its marginalization. The national mass tabloids may defend personalization and trivialization by saying that their readers turn to the television for actuality, but local papers still define themselves as a cornerstone of local democracy (Franklin and Murphy 1991; a regular theme in *UK Press Gazette*). For this to be a realistic claim, there has to be some attempt to explain the parameters of decision-making; reporting positions and reactions is not sufficient.

So why was complexity smoothed away during the middle game of the 'Save Our Homes' contest? The answer must lie in the market-place. The Nottingham *Evening Post* is well known as a Conservative-inclined paper. At the time of the controversy both the city and the county were held by Labour (and the city has since returned two more Labour MPs). Even taking the low turn-out at local elections into account, the presumption for the paper must be that there are plenty of readers or potential readers out there who can only tolerate a certain amount of overt editorial support for Conservative positions. These readers cannot be ignored: as for any local paper, advertising revenue depends upon reaching as high a proportion as possible of the local population. In order for the paper to mount a full-blooded populist campaign, the issue must be reconstructed as 'apolitical'. This is impossible if the political context and nature of the decisions involved are kept constantly in the foreground. Instead, the focus has to be shifted away from the input to the output, in this case the effect of closure. This, in turn has to be rendered such a self-evident matter that only the heartless, bureaucratic, unimaginative, rabidly political, etc. could fail to oppose it. Hence, in turn, the domestication of the issue and idealization of those against closure: residents, staff, the homes themselves – even the trade unions.

The trade union interest in keeping the homes open also served another important purpose. As we have seen, the *Evening Post* was able to argue that, if Labour-aligned unions were not blaming a Conservative government for the situation, then the Labour local politicians must be mendacious in doing so. This device, whereby the existence of political cleavages and cross-party alliances is used to construct an issue as apolitical is familiar in news media rhetoric. The more usual form is 'both sides are attacking us so we must be right/impartial/neutral'. In its new-found admiration for industrial action, the *Evening Post* failed to remember that trade unions are now forbidden in law to hold 'political strikes'. Whatever view local branches of NALGO and NUPE had of the prime cause of the closures policy, they had to focus their action entirely on their employer.

'Save Our Homes' also illustrated the very limited meaning that 'the public' has for media organizations. The only manifestations of support for the campaign seemed to be signing petitions and writing letters to the *Post*. Sources as diverse as Hall *et al.* (1978), Ericson *et al.* (1989) and Jameson (1990) all demonstrate that letters pages are not set up as a scientific sampling of public opinion, but are orchestrated into a paper's editorial line. Only those directly involved, residents and their relatives, staff and their unions, and opposed politicians, actually 'campaigned' in any meaningful sense, as far as can be detected from *Evening Post* coverage. While many Nottinghamshire citizens may have been sympathetic to the active protesters in the homes saga, they took no obvious independent initiatives.

Notwithstanding the declarations of its leader writer, the middle stage of 'Save Our Homes' was not only emotional and simplistic, but populist and party-political. For any local medium, such a strong line has commercial risks; hence the initial neutrality while alignments are formed and the forces in play assessed. It is shrewder to follow than to lead public sentiment. As the issue started to develop, the high human interest and sentimentality quotient of the issue, reinforced by union opposition, and wobbling by some members of the Labour majority on the county council, combined to make the *Evening Post* confident that it could mount an attack on the policy of closing homes, without alienating significant numbers of readers.

An even more dramatic example of local press responsiveness to opinion in its market-place occurred over the crucial coal industry. The 1984–5 miners' strike was bitter in Nottinghamshire. Most miners worked on and formed a separate union, the Union of Democratic Miners, which was consequently favoured by the Conservative government and the *Evening Post*. In the autumn of 1992, when the government proposed the virtual destruction of the British deep-mined coal industry, there was a huge and unmistakable wave of public anger manifested in national protests cutting across political parties, regions, and classes. The Nottingham *Evening Post* was very active, providing a coach for a lobby of parliament and organizing a phone-in and petition. According to the editor:

> 'We've had unquestionably the biggest response in public reaction in all the years I have been in the business, and that's more than 25. The thing about it is the unanimity of protest in Nottinghamshire. We've got Thatcherite estate agents shoulder-to-shoulder with lifelong Socialist trade unionists.'
>
> (*UK Press Gazette* 26 October 1992)

The impact of the proposed closures on Nottinghamshire and its local economy would be severe. To that extent the paper's reaction was straightforward commercial common sense, but sensitivity to political change was also demonstrated. Complex hostilities between the UDM, the NUM and the Labour Party had been shelved; Arthur Scargill had been cheered in the West End of London. No distinction could sensibly be made between the consequences for UDM-aligned Nottinghamshire and for NUM-aligned pits elsewhere: the public had indeed spoken.

This need for local media carefully to stay within range of public sentiment also explains the lack of stridency on the part of the *Post* when the closure of the elderly persons' homes was finally reversed. There may well have been party-political posturing and inept policy development during the affair, but many of the fundamental dilemmas of resources and priorities were real enough. As the *Post* editorial comment of 19 July acknowledges, there would be a cost to victory. The cash sums were large; other services would be affected as a result. When the bill was added up, it would be paid in large part by the local population, including readers of the *Evening Post*. It was time to reintroduce complexity and neutrality.

THE NEWS TREATMENT OF ELDERLY PEOPLE: WIDER IMPLICATIONS

The case studies that opened this chapter suggest that social work with elderly people is not usually national news, even when the events involve human drama or mistakes and blame. From this we can draw three important conclusions. First, problems for local authority social services departments do not always result in adverse news media treatment. This is because, second, state social work becomes news only when it is drawn into issues which feature high on the national news agenda. For all papers, but especially the mass tabloids, this includes sensational criminal trials and emotionally accessible family drama. Mid-market tabloids have a heavy investment in any event or policy that might challenge authority structures in the 'traditional' family household. The broadsheet market niche requires a regular supply of news on policy and politics. From this perspective, elderly people get news coverage in the aggregate, as the subject of legislation or as a national fiscal 'problem'. In most other respects the social construction of older people as inactive and contingent (Dant and Johnson 1991; Phillipson 1992) guarantees them the same profile in the news as other equivalent persons and groups: women; victims of crime; unemployed people; disabled people; members of ethnic communities (when not characterized as threatening social stability). All theories of news media functioning can agree on one key principle: 'news' is about the active and the holders of institutionally or symbolically powerful positions. In the west the core is the activities and interests of white, middle-aged, middle-class men; all else is periphery.

Third, national newspapers also have a financial disincentive from putting elderly people in the foreground. It is assumed that a readership in which younger, working people predominate is essential, as they are the most likely consumers of the goods advertised – although this may be mistaken given demographic and employment trends. (Further evidence for this can be adduced by a swift glance at the target groups of the constantly proliferating specialist magazine market.)

From the case studies it is, however, apparent that the very same news values and commercial pressures may cause elderly people to feature in local news media. Formal power structures, target consumers, and identification are measured on very different scales. The closure of a home might affect the mother of a workmate or neighbour, or the job of an old friend of your sister from schooldays. Or your friend may have met a friend of his in the pub who knows a councillor who claims to have tasty inside information. Having ceased to be about the impact of abstract policy on unknown elderly people, the same issues become interesting, readable – and saleable.

We have seen that the Nottinghamshire elderly persons' home saga was never 'social work news'. It is not difficult to imagine circumstances in which similar events could be constructed in terms of social work practice and policies, with senior officers cast as lead villains. This would obviously be professionally difficult and personally painful for those involved. It is a mistake, though, to allow this constant risk to social work professionals to be treated as analogous with freak weather, where the only hope is battening down the hatches and waiting until it has passed. The news treatment of the elderly residents, although saccharine and oversimplified on this occasion, suggests extensive possibilities for presenting local authority social services as doing good work which mostly satisfies users, and with which the local community can identify. Attempts to gain positive news coverage need not collude with images of residents in homes as pathetically grateful, or passive recipients of local charity visits. Users of domiciliary services might be willing to feature, alongside staff, in accounts of the satisfactions and problems of trying to retain an independent community-based life.

For the chair of Nottinghamshire Social Services Committee, it must have been hard to detect any difference in the *Evening Post*'s treatment from '"going for the jugular"' or being '"crucified"'. But it is important to note that the paper's attack was not permanent. Local politicians crucially depend upon local media – as the 'Save Our Homes' affair vividly demonstrated – but local media also need local politicians. Constructing local news consists largely of maintaining contact with those persons and organizations that form the local institutional order. Indeed, as we have seen, the stated mission of local media often goes well beyond this to claims that they are themselves a vital means of maintaining the structure, whether by providing stocks for the wrongdoer or praise for the worthy. (As an illustration of the former, the only other item on the same page as the first *Evening Post* 'special report' on the homes closure plan was a complete column 'In the courts'. This is not big-time crime: one defendant was fined £25.00 for 'exceeding axle weight'.)

As Franklin and Murphy (1991) point out, local newspapers implicitly, and sometimes explicitly, embrace a functionalist notion of the organic community and body politic. For this reason, persons and power structures may be attacked, but in ritualized and ultimately restrained terms. As well as the philosophy, there is also the mundane practical requirement of keeping working relationships with local contacts. So there are rich possibilities, and larger political imperatives, for professional social work staff to follow the local party politicians and exploit the symbiotic relationship between the local media and local government in a more pro-active and organized way. This does not mean that 'bad news' could – or should – be suppressed. But, as writers in social work's own trade press show in Chapter 7, skilful and truthful damage limitation is certainly possible, as is the frank promotion of 'good news' in local news media. This is a message already received and acted upon by the probation service, as we shall see in the following chapter.

Chapter 5

Courting coverage – probation and the press

The challenge in scrutinizing the press coverage of the probation service is not interpreting the message, but finding that coverage in the first place. While local authority social services staff appear to yearn for a media-free world, the probation service is trying to raise its profile in the news. The search for news media visibility is being pursued both nationally, through organizations like NAPO and the Association of Chief Officers of Probation (ACOP), and locally. By mid-1991 about a quarter of probation services had a full-time external/public relations officer; nearly all the remaining areas had an officer who had PR as a part of their responsibility.

None of the chapters in Franklin and Parton's (1991) review of social work's relations with the news media discuss the probation service. Articles about media relations in the probation press are rare. One of the few examples (Smyth 1990) is about promoting the Greater Manchester Service. It is written in a wry but cheerful tone very different from the social services equivalents. Is this because probation work is not social work? Not according to many in the service itself, who characterize its work precisely as social work within the criminal justice system, nor to a *Daily Mail* editorial (29 February 1992) which comments, with manifest distaste, that 'four fifths of officers' training is devoted to social work'.

Surely the probation service shares many of the characteristics used to explain the allegedly poor public image of social work felt so acutely by its practitioners? It often appears to take a radical stance, advocating both non-common-sense explanations of offending which challenge models of individual responsibility, and hare-brained non-punitive responses to offenders. (On 23 March 1992 Independent Television News described a two-year probation order as 'going free'.) Nor is probation work a 'traditional' profession: it falls into that group, along with local authority social workers and teachers, whose clients are provided by the state

(Johnson 1972). Those clients are axiomatically society's outcasts, having been convicted of a criminal offence, so probation officers are 'contaminated' by their dealings with them. Worse, their 'professional association', NAPO, is actually a full-blooded trade union that sounds off against government policy and has conferences that take political correctness in language and demeanour very seriously indeed.

Few members of the public have direct contact with social services. This ignorance of its powers, structure and practices is shared by many news media workers (Fry 1991; Golding and Middleton 1982) and is often cited as a reason for the potential power of negative media coverage. Only first-hand or trusted second-hand knowledge provides the confidence to qualify or dismiss media accounts (Philo 1990). Is not the probation service in an even weaker position, hidden from view, trying to do good to undeserving criminals?

It can hardly be claimed that the probation service is working in a non-newsworthy area. Crime has always been a staple of the news media (Chibnall 1977; Ericson *et al.* 1987; Schlesinger *et al.* 1991; Soothill and Walby 1991). As we have seen, two of the most influential studies of the UK media, Cohen's (1973) book defining the 'moral panic', and its reinterpretation within a class analysis by Hall and his colleagues (1978), use crime and the criminal justice system as their empirical core. More recently, Ericson *et al.*'s blockbusting three-volume series on Canadian press and television work (1987; 1989; 1991) focuses on crime and 'control agencies' – although the Canadian equivalent of probation is not included. At an everyday level, a glance through any newspaper, broadsheet or tabloid, national or local, will show that criminal offences, court proceedings and the effects of crime and the criminal justice system are all given significant space. Only the detail, mix and style vary with the type of newspaper. Crime and detective series have long been the dominant genre of popular UK television drama. They are now being joined by a proliferation of actuality/reconstruction programmes in the mould of *Crimewatch UK* (usefully examined by Schlesinger *et al.* 1991).

Why is the probation service behaving more like one of the big social work charities than a part of state social work? Ironically, the answer lies in its relationship to government. Although still organized on a local basis, 80 per cent of the funding for the service comes from central government and is thus in direct competition with other calls on public funds. Probation is struggling for resources with law enforcement rivals like the prison service, large voluntary organizations, and even HM Customs and Excise, as Schlesinger and his colleagues (1991) demonstrate. Throughout the 1980s the Thatcher Conservative government identified itself as strong on law and order. (See Hale 1992 for a very useful review of social trends, political response and legislative change.) Towards the end of the decade, however, it was clear that the cost of imprisonment was becoming insupportable. 'Punishment in the community' had to be recast as a suitable penalty for a higher proportion of non-violent offenders. While the probation service was the obvious agency to manage this, a succession of informal and official pronouncements from mid-1988 onwards contained the clear message that the service must toughen up both methods and image or be marginalized at best.

An early indication of government thinking is an article in *The Times* (7 March 1988) by John Patten, then a minister in the Home Office. He focuses particularly on the adverse effect of prison on young offenders:

> But if we are to persuade the public that it is worth – and safe – looking beyond punishment in prison to 'punishment in the community' we *must* be able to increase the degree of discipline and control exerted on an offender.
>
> (*The Times* 7 March 1988; emphasis in original)

The same themes are prominent in the Green Paper (Cm 424 1988) published the following July. Three objectives are identified for community disposals: punishment by restriction of freedom; reduction of further offending; and reparation/compensation. 'It is also important that the probation service should demonstrate to judges and magistrates the work which the service is doing with serious offenders' (Cm 424 1988: para. 2.13). Should the probation service fail to get the message, the Green Paper includes a discussion of setting up a new agency to supervise 'punishment in the community'. Addressing ACOP's annual conference that year (*The Times* 16 September 1988), John Patten maintained the mix of threats and blandishments: '"We do need to develop exciting and new ways of punishing in the community those who commit less serious crimes ... The probation service must come to terms with the idea of punishment and control as well as helping and reforming."' There is also a strong hint that presentational changes are an important part of the strategy: 'Most people in the world outside probation quite naturally use words like "punishment", "control", "tough and demanding". They prefer "offender" to "client". They are surprised when probation officers do not and the seeds of confusion are sown.'

Not that the service could confine itself to a higher profile and more abrasive terminology. In 1990 a further Green Paper (Cm 965 1990) was published as a companion to the White Paper (Cm 966 1990) which formed the basis of the 1991 Criminal Justice Act. The theme of the Green Paper is control, not only of offenders by probation officers, but of officers by management and the courts, of management by the probation committee, of local services by a strengthened inspectorate plus Home Office appointments to local committees, and by a number of further possible measures, including 100 per cent government funding and the formation of a national service for England and Wales.

For the probation service, therefore, the struggle joined in 1988 continues. It must contrive to persuade central government and sentencers that it is sufficiently controlling, that it is efficient, that it provides value for money, etc. – and that these objectives can be maintained by the existing decentralized, semi-autonomous system. It must also persuade government that the public is being convinced of these qualities. Yet many within the service remain strongly committed to probation as work in the interests of clients too. For very different reasons, then, the government and the service are agreed that a higher public profile is needed for probation work.

Using the same approach as that applied to the press treatment of social services work, I examined a number of instances of probation in the press. These were not only well-known 'scandals', but also apparently similar cases which did not attract equivalent attention. I also interviewed several agency staff dealing with external/public relations work, and analysed a sample of news releases and press cuttings relating to ACOP, NAPO and a local probation service.

Any attempt at news management has two lines of action: to contain adverse unsolicited coverage and to try to create the conditions for favourable media treatment. The rest of this chapter will fall, therefore, into three parts: the first will review the extent to which the probation service receives unsolicited news coverage. Next I shall consider some aspects of pro-active news management by NAPO, ACOP and two probation services. The final section will analyse the extent and character of unsolicited probation news, and its implications for the strategies being adopted to 'place' news.

PROBATION IN THE PRESS

During May, June and July 1991 I collected the Nottingham city edition of the Nottingham *Evening Post*. Over that period, the probation service was the subject of only one item. Under a large headline 'Probation staff in work ban' (1 May 1991), the paper reported the start of national industrial action against 'a substantial increase in unsocial hours'. The style is of a neutral news item, but only NAPO's perspective is reported, so there is neither direct nor indirect criticism of probation officers. The relative silence of the *Evening Post* is interesting. It is not a left-of-centre paper and the Nottinghamshire Probation Service is well known to be at the liberal end of the probation service continuum. It cannot be that there is no probation news, as it receives news releases from the local service. Maybe criminal justice is not an editorial priority. Incidental evidence for this emerged during a scrutiny of news items published in response to news releases produced by the National Association for the Care and Resettlement of Offenders (NACRO) during June 1991. The *Evening Post* did not appear to have taken up any of the issues. In contrast, one NACRO statement, on the level of prison overcrowding, was used by at least thirty local papers.

So what does probation have to do to get into the news? Is its 'bad news' more likely to be picked up? An incident, which the *Guardian* (22 May 1985) headlined 'Judge scorns probation officer's pleas for "brute"', looked promising. A woman probation officer had written in a report that a man convicted of grievous bodily harm on his three-month-old son needed the '"on-going support of the probation service"'. Lord Justice Lawton did not agree: '"In a long career on the bench I have never heard such rubbish. What this man needs is punishment – he is a brute".' Taking examples from the upmarket, mid-market and mass-selling tabloid UK daily press showed that neither *The Times*, nor the *Daily Mirror* reported the case at all. The *Sun* and the *Daily Express*, neither noted for editorial support of state social work, limited their coverage to brief items on p. 7 and p. 15 respectively. Both identified the probation officer as a woman and quoted phrases from the report which are clearly intended to make the reader scoff at her advocacy of wet psychological explanations for wickedness. However, neither paper widened the argument to the service as a whole nor was it taken up in feature or editorial comment, although it would seem to fit neatly into the 'wimp' stereotype of the social worker summed up by Franklin and Parton (1991).

Significantly, the inventory of social workers as young, inexperienced and gullible was being refined, according to Franklin and Parton (1991), at precisely this historical period. Three of the court cases which sparked major controversies in and about social work practice – Jasmine Beckford, Tyra Henry and Kimberley Carlile – took place between 1985 and 1987.

After the conviction of Andrew Neil for Tyra Henry's murder, it emerged that an internal report of Lambeth Social Services had criticized, *inter alia*, the probation service (*Guardian* 26 July 1985). Neil had been on licence and yet the probation service was not included in the sweeping and vitriolic accounts of social work ineptitude in the news coverage of the case by mid-market and mass tabloid papers described in Chapter 2.

During the Charlene Salt trial (see Chapter 2) it emerged, as we have seen, that an array of health and welfare professionals had been involved with the family. Yet it is only by reading the Oldham *Evening Chronicle* (24 October 1985) that one discovers, as an incidental detail, that the accused was on probation. While this could not have been taken up during the trial, it is an angle on the case which none of the national papers highlighted in their review after the verdict. Not only was the probation service not criticized, it was not even mentioned in a scenario where the multiplicity of professions involved was one of the most salient features of both the case and the news stories, particularly in the *Daily Mirror*.

The *Sun*, as it often tells us, is Britain's biggest selling newspaper. It is Conservative-supporting, pro-police and anti-gay, and wages war on 'bungling bureaucrats'. (See Chippindale and Horrie (1990) for an account of the *Sun*'s preoccupations.) Surely, then, there could have been grist for the news mill in a furore over criticisms by two probation officers of a poster in a Hartlepool police station which showed people alleged to have AIDS. The two officers were suspended (and subsequently disciplined – although not for expressing their disquiet but for failing to pursue it through the mechanisms laid down in probation service policy). The row widened: NAPO threatened a 'no confidence' motion in the CPO; the CPO was criticized by the chair of Cleveland Social Services; local MPs became involved, etc. The imbroglio attracted very extensive local press coverage in the Cleveland area during June and July 1991, including news items and features on the unfolding drama, and editorial comment. Among the national press, only *The Independent* reported the affair, focusing on the civil liberties implications both for people with AIDS and for the two officers. Neither the *Guardian*, which specializes in this type of news, nor the *Daily Telegraph*, which is distinctive for the volume of its news stories, reported the issue. Nor did the mid-market and popular tabloids take up the possible AIDS and 'local do-gooders fall out' angles. Not even the magic word 'Cleveland' raised a response.

While it can be argued that the intersection of civil rights and public policy is not likely to generate major treatment in the mass tabloids, surely a court case about alleged sex abuse where the accused is a probation officer with strongly held religious views would score on a number of *Sun* rating scales? Apparently not, as the only national newspaper (and this categorization is itself debatable) to report the case in July 1991 was the *Sport*, despite extensive local coverage throughout the five-day hearing, culminating in emotional scenes after the probation officer's acquittal.

Among the many criminal justice initiatives taken by the Conservative government in the 1980s was the importation from the US of electronic 'tagging' of offenders. An apparently progressive, government-sponsored, 'solution' to a major social problem, featuring gee-whizz technology would surely be given favourable treatment in most of the national press. By extension, its opponents would be criticized. When the scheme was launched by the Home Office in May 1989, both NAPO and NACRO were very hostile. Examination of the cuttings collected by NACRO in response to its news release showed a bifurcation in the press treatment. Of the tabloids, only the *Daily Mail* (9 May 1989) mentioned tagging at all. Its critics were simply not reported. Several of the broadsheets covered the issue, as did a number of regional and local dailies. A number of them used NAPO as an 'authorized knower' to provide the 'against' case for balance in hard news format. Again, there was no adverse comment on NAPO's stance.

One of the most anguished complaints by social workers about their press coverage is that in the highly publicized child murder trials failure to prevent the child's death seemed to be put on a footing with committing the crime itself (see Franklin and Parton 1991). Elements of this process are certainly prominent in the saturation coverage given to the conclusion of the Colin Evans/Marie Payne case in December 1984. Evans, who had a record of convictions for sexual assault over the previous seventeen years, was sentenced to thirty years' imprisonment for the sexual assault and murder of a 4-year-old girl. The case was covered by all the national newspapers. The *Sun* (five pages) and the *Daily Star* (nearly six pages) gave it most prominence, with wide-ranging features obviously prepared well in advance, underscoring Soothill and Walby's (1991: 35) observation that crime is the only topic in which the mass tabloids undertake activity resembling 'investigative reporting'. (They further observe, however, that this does not usually extend to questioning the police 'script', but consists mostly of descriptive background material within the paradigm already established.)

Marie Payne lived and died in Essex, while Evans lived in Reading, Berkshire. During the trial Evans's history emerged, including a number of previously undiscovered sexual assaults on children and confirmation that he had committed assaults of which he had been previously acquitted. Evans had been introduced to Toc H (a Christian voluntary organization) by a Berkshire senior probation officer who did not tell Toc H about Evans's record. While at Toc H, Evans had established himself in a position to allocate tasks and set up a babysitting organization. He then worked with families referred by social services without any checks into his history, because of the respectability conferred by Toc H. This aspect of the case attracted most attention: 'THIS MAN LET SEX FIEND BE A BABYSITTER' ran a three-deck headline of 2.5 cm type across two pages of the *Sun*'s '3–page dossier' (18 December 1984), beside a large picture of the officer looking bewildered and distressed.

The news treatment of the case included five elements, their weight and balance depending on the particular newspaper: the offence itself; Evans's history; the pain caused to the families involved; the culpability of individuals; system/policy failures on the part of the police, the probation service and social services. As could be predicted, all the mid-market and mass tabloids focused on personalization and titillation, with details of the offences, interviews with the families, and material on Evans's background. Where these features attempted to explain his behaviour, they fell into the psychopathological model of the 'sex-fiend' described by Soothill and Walby (1991). Such abnormals, it was implied, should be obvious to the skilled observer – a frame of reference parallel to some of the other trials following the death of a child examined in Chapter 2. Failure to prevent the offences was thus a matter of personal inadequacy or worse, with the greatest blame attaching to the probation officer, described as a 'bungler' by the *Sun* (18 December 1984) using one of its favourite terms of abuse.

The use of pictures is a telling index of the editorial assessment of the key elements in a news story. Only *The Times*, the *Daily Telegraph* and the *Morning Star* did not include a picture of the probation officer.

Among the 'catalogue of blunders' (*Daily Telegraph* headline, 18 December 1984) were a number of failures by the police during the four-teen months between Marie Payne's disappearance and the discovery of her body. The attention given to these is not totally predictable: they were detailed by the *Sun* (with some prominence – but then that precious commodity, a *Sun* reader, had supplied some crucial missed evidence), *The Times*, the *Daily Star* and the *Daily Telegraph*, but not by the *Daily Mirror* or the *Daily Mail*. The *Daily Express* neutralized the issue by an offsetting account of the 'alert policeman' who led to Evans's arrest.

Rather than the dreadful error of judgement on the part of the probation officer, the continuing significance of the Colin Evans case was the failure of inter-agency liaison and the subsequent setting up of a system for checking the criminal record, if any, of persons undertaking unsupervised work with children. These system/policy aspects of the case were given as much space as other issues in the *Guardian* and the *Daily*

Telegraph, but – surprisingly – relatively little in *The Times*. The mass tabloids' short-lived attention to the policy implications came through follow-up items the next day, as the issue moved into the political arena of MPs' demands for the setting up of a register of sex offenders and for the dismissal of the probation officer.

Three newspapers had editorial comments on the case on 18 December: the *Daily Mail*, the *Daily Express* and the *Daily Star*. The *Star* criticizes past parole decisions, 'a probation officer' and 'a social worker' in general terms, but puts its main emphasis on access to the records of sex offenders. The *Daily Express* editorial concludes 'The police might also like to explain why it took so long to catch Evans . . . But the most urgent questions are for the "caring" professionals. This case suggests appalling laxity – of practice and of thought.' (Earlier on the writer had suggested 'criminal negligence charges' might be appropriate.)

The widest net of blame is cast by the *Daily Mail*. The courts are criticized for 'scandalous leniency'; 'And the probation officer concerned? Sacked? You only have to ask the question to know the answer: Reprimanded.' The second part of the editorial links the Evans case to the conviction of a London supply (temporary replacement) teacher for supplying drugs. 'Our courts, our probation and social services, our schools and education authorities cannot toy tolerantly with violators and corrupters of youth.' Most of the rest of the page is given over to a feature, the main message of which is that London supply teachers are predominantly failures and misfits – with a caricature illustration of a loony left teacher, replete with badges supporting CND and the (then current) miners' strike.

Another demonstration of the distinctive world view of the *Daily Mail* is a news item of 12 April 1991, apparently based on a Home Office news release about 'the Government's determination to make punishment in the community an alternative to overcrowded jails'.

> [The minister] said yesterday that for the first time probation officers would be brought into the centre of the criminal justice system. Over the next three years the probation service would receive extra money amounting to 25 per cent above the inflation rate and 800 extra staff would be employed.
>
> (*Daily Mail* 12 April 1991)

But the headline and opening paragraph? 'Lenient probation officers may end up in court'; 'Probation officers who do not supervise young criminals properly could be taken to court for failing their duty.'

In the coverage of the Colin Evans/Marie Payne case a probation officer is named, pictured and blamed and his dismissal demanded. Although this fits very well with the presentational and discursive framework applied to major social services child death controversies, its significance for probation-related news is that it is – to date – unique.

ACTIVELY SEEKING COVERAGE

How does the probation service try to get useful news coverage? At the national level, ACOP is limited by the small number of probation services and consequently has very limited resources. In the struggle for media attention the Association does not yet seem to have established itself as an authorized knower, routinely to be contacted for intelligence or reactions to events. Between January and June 1991 ACOP issued fifteen news releases. Six resulted in coverage, almost all in the national broadsheet press. In only one instance was ACOP quoted as the sole expert voice. In seven newspaper articles some combination of NAPO, NACRO, the Prison Reform Trust, and the Howard League had been used instead to comment on matters which had been the subject of an ACOP news release. NACRO exists to influence penal policy; in purely material terms it and the other large pressure groups are formidable occupants of limited territory.

NAPO has had an officer responsible for external relations since 1984; the union reacted to the policy events of 1988 by making his role much more active. As well as parliamentary lobbying, public speaking and producing publications, he solicits news coverage through news releases. About four or five a year reflect major NAPO policy initiatives; the rest are shorter position statements or reactions to events, an overall total of about twenty per year. It is clear that, unlike ACOP, NAPO is well established as a reliable media contact for news and comment. In the year to May 1992, all its news releases received at least one national press mention. Some were covered in national and local papers, and national and local broadcast media as well. Topics included curbs on people on bail, NAPO's hostility to privatized prisons, its evidence to the Royal Commission on Criminal Justice, violence in hostels, and prison conditions. NAPO also routinely receives several phone calls every day asking for background material or comment on current issues. About four-fifths of these calls are from national news media.

One of NAPO's most successful campaigns to date was a news release in March 1992, following up its earlier assertion that there might be 700 innocent people in jail in England and Wales. This resulted in prominent coverage in seven national papers, news and features on national and regional television, national and local radio items, and local/regional press accounts. *The Independent*, which is one of the most regular users of NAPO's placed news (the other is the *Guardian*), gave it a large double column placing, illustrated with a montage of photograph plus graphics.

National press use of NAPO as a source of background information and comment is directly related to the newspaper's general editorial investment in professional and policy issues. The right-wing broadsheets make contact less often than the centre left, the tabloids very rarely (with the exception of the *Daily Mail* and occasionally the *Daily Mirror*).

One local probation service with a full-time public relations officer (PRO) is in the south-west of England. His activities include producing a relatively glossy annual report, editing a twice-yearly newsletter, disseminating news releases, responding to media enquiries and collecting/circulating a weekly digest of press cuttings about probation and criminal justice issues. Local media are supplied with information on both local initiatives and major national policy developments. The officer sees an important part of his role as forming good working relationships with journalists – easier with some than others because of their personal style of operation, regardless of their employer. A specific example of the value of such trust was an agreement to delay publicity about a serious incident at a bail hostel for twenty-four hours, with the quid pro quo of an informative response from the service at the end of that period.

The papers clipped by the PRO include the national broadsheet and mid-market papers, and all the local and regional paid-for papers. Mentions of the area in local papers elsewhere are forwarded by ACOP. (Neither the local PRO, NAPO, the Home Office, nor ACOP clip the mass tabloids.) An analysis of the cuttings collected during August, September and October 1991 yielded thirty-six items on the local area, three of which were in the national media: one was favourable, one neutral and one negative (the *Daily Express* picking up an attack by a local Tory councillor on a 'crackpot' scheme to give driving lessons to young offenders). Of the thirty-three local press items, thirty were neutral or positive about the probation service. As an example of a neutral item: a local doctor attacked sentencing sex offenders to probation. His criticisms were of the bench and the article was set up in standard 'impartial' news format with plenty of space given to a probation service reply. Positive coverage included an account of a successful victim support scheme and stories with pictures of promoted probation officers.

As far as it was possible to tell from the text, about twenty of the positive items arose from probation service PR work, both news releases and the annual report. Some of the remaining approving coverage came from Home Office, police or NACRO PR work. Only three clippings were wholly negative, two from an aggressively populist local Sunday paper (and one of these seemed to be based on the *Daily Express* item above). The other was a diary item in a normally friendly regional daily ridiculing the concern about 'correct' language at the 1991 NAPO conference. This was presumably picked up from the national press, which had gleefully covered a sub-committee report leaked to the press, despite union attempts to keep it as an internal document. 'TALK IS CHEAP FATSO' was the *Daily Mirror* (15 October 1991) headline about 'Conference delegates . . . on the lookout for discrimination against just about everything'. (It was also covered in the *Daily Telegraph* and the *Daily Mail* but with heavy irony rather than vitriol.)

The situation in a Midlands probation service provides an example of an area without a full-time PR appointment. Here an officer allocates 25 per cent of his time to PR. He fields media approaches, subject to consultation with management on sensitive and/or political issues; produces news releases, mostly directed at the local paid-for evening paper or, to a lesser extent, local radio and even less to local free-sheets; publishes a tri-annual newsletter, very similar to that of the south-western service discussed above. He does not compile an annual report, as the service management has concluded that they are not effective in communicating with the media. Asked about local media take-up, the officer's estimate was 'about 80 per cent', usually involving a request for further information. In about a fifth to a quarter of instances the local paper would use a news release as the basis of a feature. Occasionally he sends items to the national media. Material on the relationship between poverty and offending had been taken up by some of the national broadsheets. On the other hand, the officer is keenly aware that, lacking personal relationships with newsgatherers and any sense of loyalty to the area, the outcome can be very unpredictable or at least – as Smyth (1990) also described – not what the service had intended. An item about a successful campaign to improve payments for a lodgings scheme was transformed by the *Sun* into a tale about '£80 a week for sex fiend'.

A similarly salutary experience of how news media gather in and reinterpret material arose in Northumbria, where the Chief Probation Officer had commissioned an internal report (Northumbria Probation Service 1992) on the lessons that might be learned from the civil unrest in parts of his area in the summer of 1991. The final version was to be made public with a covering news release. Having taken it to the ACOP conference in draft form, the CPO gave a copy to a BBC Radio 4 reporter. The following day (28 February 1992) a brief account was broadcast, picking out the eighth and final 'reflection on the role of the probation service' – which had been identified in the report as 'perhaps the most important'. For a variety of reasons to do with more 'high risk' offenders, the government's policy on '"punishment in the community"', and a change in styles of work to 'set programmes and scripts', the service had little direct knowledge of the Meadowell estate, the main focus of the disturbances (Northumbria Probation Service 1992: 10). (The other seven points included observations on the realities of life for non-offenders; the 'racial dimension to the disturbances'; loss of experienced staff; increasing workloads; the lack of pro-active work with the news media during the disturbances; the need for monitoring work with police and courts; and the lack of any predesigned 'response plan' to the demands made by the disturbances.)

The day after the Radio 4 news item the report was taken up by five national papers: *The Times*, the *Daily Telegraph*, *The Independent*, the *Daily Mail*, and the *Daily Express*. All followed the Radio 4 interpretation and developed only the 'desk-bound' theme – not at all the same as 'office-bound' for probation officers, but perhaps so for journalists! The broadsheets all used further comment from the CPO about the context of government policy and the need to be '"more visible"' (*Daily Telegraph* 29 February 1992). While the report is characterized as critical, and the CPO described as 'admitting' its findings (for example, *Daily Telegraph* 29 February 1992), their treatment allows the probation service to define what remains of the issue.

The *Daily Express* is both briefer and more confused: 'Officers' leader Harry Fletcher claimed the Home Office told his men [*sic*] to stay inside.' This is, presumably, a condensed version of a NAPO comment on a sentence in the report: 'At the height of the disturbances probation officers were advised against home visiting' (Northumbria Probation Service 1992: 5).

As on other occasions, it was the *Daily Mail* that enlarged the issue most, both conceptually and literally, with a library picture, the largest headline and leader comment. The substance of the news item resembles that in other papers but the leader uses the 'ignorant plus deskbound' theme as a springboard. The decline of community links is 'ironic', it writes, because it was these that were used by the service to resist government proposals for a national service. This conceptual leap is achieved by rather disingenuously eliding 'local' as home/neighbourhood with 'local' as local government area-based. Calling it an 'isolated bureaucracy', the final paragraph suddenly announces:

Moreover, four fifths of officers' training is devoted to social work and only a fifth to criminal justice. This balance is wrong. The first duty of probation staff, in Tyneside or anywhere else, should be to ensure that the orders of the court are observed.

(Daily Mail 29 February 1992)

In this rhetorically skilled paragraph the opening and closing sentences are put in opposition by the unargued and metaphorical declaration on 'balance'. As a result of this device, being trained in social work is made somehow to entail failing to enforce the orders of the court.

INTERPRETING THE NEWS TREATMENT OF PROBATION WORK

Reviewing the evidence on unsolicited coverage we have seen that the probation service rarely has to undertake damage limitation in response to hostile news media attention in the way that local authority social services see as a constant possibility. This is not because the service is never drawn into situations where there is a hue and cry about attributing blame, as the Tyra Henry and Charlene Salt cases illustrate.

The media reaction to the Colin Evans/Marie Payne case, on the other hand, strongly resembled the treatment of child murder cases which have raised questions about social services. Here was a man well known to the criminal justice system over many years who was able to continue offending through a combination of his skilful manipulation of the system, bad judgements by professionals, poor inter-agency liaison, and unimaginative police procedures. In their different ways both the tabloid and broadsheet accounts of the case spin a large web of uncomfortable questions about who should have done what and when. How then to achieve 'closure'? In the Colin Evans case two responses were distilled: make sex offenders' records available and sack the person who made the most visible mistake. That this mistake had probably enabled Evans to continue his history of sexual abuse, but could not be directly linked with the murder, mirrors those accounts of social services cases where social workers seem to be held responsible for the crime itself. (See Franklin and Parton (1991) and preceding chapters for instances.) There are, though, a number of important respects in which the media treatment of the probation officer/service in the Colin Evans case did not fit the 'social worker to blame' template. That the officer was a 54-year-old man with twenty years' experience restricted the application of stereotypes. Having disciplined him, the local service seems to have closed ranks very effectively. Only the CPO was quoted and then he refused to elaborate beyond a formal statement. The officer himself was quoted directly by one paper. Unlike some of the most acrimonious child death and child abuse cases, no public division of opinion emerged between the main agencies involved – despite the potential for mutual accusation. Was this because of a well-organized media strategy, or because the newsgatherers approached the probation service with greater deference as part of the criminal justice system rather than part of the rough-and-tumble of local politics? Moreover, despite the vilification poured on the probation officer, the press coverage did not at any stage widen this out to either the Berkshire Probation Service or the *idea* of probation work, in the way that has occurred in social services *causes célèbres*.

Within social work, the probation service is often said to be more 'professional' than local authority social services. The explanation most frequently proffered is that it borrows social status from the courts. It is said to have the further advantages that it has for a long time been all-qualified, and that the service's task is simpler to define and thus its successes easier to demonstrate. This perspective is located in an unarticulated version of the idealist model of the professions described in Chapter 8, in which at least partly autonomous occupational groups are thought to have social standing in direct proportion to the distinctiveness of their cognitive knowledge. In reality, the probation service is no less a creature of central government than local authority social services – arguably more so, given the financial regime. Its knowledge base and expertise are entirely contingent on the activities determined for it under statute.

However one defines 'profession', though, being a pressure group has always been part of the concept – even before 'pressure group politics' expanded exponentially. In this respect, the probation service is much better placed than the rest of state social work. Its mission, as laid out in the 'Requirements for Probation Training in the Diploma in Social Work in England and Wales' (CCETSW 1991: Annex 2) is clear and easily grasped (even if less easy to achieve). Objectives like 'provide the courts with a range of effective community-based disposals' and 'supervise offenders within the community' are even capable of the kind of performance measures now imposed throughout the public sector. From the bounded task and relatively small size of the service as a whole comes the kind of solidarity and potential for unified action undreamed of in local authority social services. Chief Probation Officers are so few that they all know each other well – although this does not guarantee concerted action, as ACOP demonstrates. NAPO, too, has a level of policy co-ordination and a capacity to respond to events beyond the ability of both BASW and NALGO for their different reasons.

Dealing with offenders may, paradoxically, remove the problem of working at the social deviancy frontier. As Parton has persuasively argued (1991: 60, 141), over the last decade the driving force of public policy in child protection work, as in mental health work and the whole field of social benefits, has been to limit costs by targeting activity at a residuum so 'dangerous' or inadequate that it must be controlled in the interests of social stability. When local authority social workers advocate the rights of clients to benefits and services, they are working directly against this by attempting to enlarge the category of the 'deserving poor', with all its fiscal implications. Probation officers, however progressive in their explanations of offending behaviour and humane in their methods of dealing with it, are not challenging definitions, but debating solutions. They are seen to be on the side of 'us', in dealing with a deviant (for now) 'them', defined elsewhere.

Not only is the probation service able to conceptualize and demonstrate 'success' but there is less likelihood of being held to account for 'failure'. One might consider that supervising a parolee presents the same risk of blame for the client's actions as working with parents suspected of violence. But probation's clients are already classified as deviant. If they complete their probation successfully, it is the officer's success. If the client re-offends or otherwise falters, it is that client's responsibility. The service does not have to identify the 'monster', only contain.

The relative media invisibility of probation work is, though, not to be understood only in terms of the content of the job. The service as an institutional site does not fit with newsgathering values and routines. In terms of national daily papers, probation officers are not key players in the judicial process. Their work before sentence is inaccessible. In most criminal cases press interest in the defendant(s) ends on sentence, particularly in the tabloids. The few exceptions, as Soothill and Walby (1991) point out, are sensational cases. In these, probation or other community-based penalties are unlikely disposals. The broadsheets sometimes report on probation issues as a small part of their concern with policy and politics, but even here the experience of NAPO and ACOP show most of the attention comes from the non-Tory papers.

Locally the probation service will not be on regular 'newsbeats' unless local PR efforts have actively built the contact. Its committee meetings are private; it does not produce party political set pieces; it needs no electoral platform; and significant costs do not fall directly on the local population. It cannot, therefore, be transformed into the local politics which is such a central component of local news production, as we have seen in the discussion of the Nottinghamshire elderly persons' homes affair in Chapter 5.

In relation to the probation service, as over other social work issues, both statutory and voluntary, the *Daily Mail* is *sui generis* (except for the paler version of the same agenda produced by the *Daily Express*). Unlike other media it explicitly identifies the service as social work, and applies its customary frame of reference.

THE PROSPECTS FOR PROBATION NEWS MANAGEMENT

The probation service has two objectives in its self-promotion activities: to influence opinion-formers over resources and policies, and to encourage the public at large to accept community disposals. Paradoxically, local media rather than the mass national press have been chosen as the vehicle to reach the wider public – undoubtedly a rational choice. For these, the main criterion of news will be local identification, so even 'good news' is news (see Chapter 1). Drama and conflict seem less vital than in national media. Controversial issues are usually treated with the delicacy that comes from not wanting to alienate a large section of your consumers, as we have seen with both the Nottingham *Evening Post* and the *Leicester Mercury* (over the Frank Beck case). There is the possibility of making good personal contacts among local newsgatherers.

Even when local services try to get national publicity, part of the aim may well be to reach local influentials: judges, the bench, senior police, other agencies, etc. Appearing in the broadsheet press confers that extra dimension of credibility. This is also the audience for the local 'newsletters' produced by both the services discussed above; they are not intended for clients or the wider public.

Financial pressure on both print and broadcast media has increased the likelihood that cheap, 'placed' news will at least be considered (Franklin and Murphy 1991). This does not apply only to campaigns by individual probation services: local radio take-up of NAPO news releases suggests that local radio and regional television news may be the best way to mobilize popular support where this is part of the policy objective, as in the NAPO campaign over miscarriages of justice. The largest selling national dailies, paradoxically, are the least effective vehicle for reaching 'the public' because of their lack of interest in process and abstract policy issues.

Most attempts to get national publicity, however, are aimed at neither the public nor local worthies, but at national opinion-formers and policy-makers in government, the judiciary and other sections of the criminal justice system: the 'policy community' (Schlesinger *et al.* 1991, quoting Kingdon 1984). The target media are the national broadsheet press and television current affairs programmes. In the competition for political priority the stakes are high. Other contestants include heavyweights like the police and established, well-resourced pressure groups such as NACRO. Some of these, for example the Prison Reform Trust, do not dissipate their resources by attempting to persuade 'the public' at all. Even small pressure groups may be, as Schlesinger and colleagues (1991) point out, very well connected.

Both locally and nationally the crucial resource is staff time, which is hard to justify against front-line work. The probation service has a range of compelling reasons for keeping its locally based organization and funding, but there is little doubt that this reduces its potential effect-iveness in the centralized world of political and single-interest pressure group lobbying, especially given the almost completely London-centred field of vision of the national news media. On the other hand, the lack of adverse publicity (always excepting the *Daily Mail*) suggests that the probation service has both an advantageous institutional location and considerable cultural 'capital' to draw on with the public and opinion-formers, provided its concerns can be packaged to fit news media formats and agendas.

In the 1970s, to contain growing fiscal pressures, the definition of poverty had to be narrowed. Some of the poor had to be reclassified as 'undeserving' – and thus deviant. Golding and Middleton (1982) write of the ease with which the concept was resurrected and reinserted into public discourse. This was achieved, they argue, by mobilizing an enduring individualist tradition demonstrated by centuries of punitive legislation, and further facilitated by the individualist professional value system of newsgatherers and processors. To solve the equivalent fiscal problems created by criminal deviance, an apparently contrary – but actually identical – process is under way. Some of those previously classified as a danger must be redefined as not dangerous, but suitable for 'punishment in the community'. The remaining hard core of the 'really dangerous' will be those who 'need' to be incarcerated. The process exactly parallels the search for the 'dangerous' person and family in contemporary child protection practice (Parton 1991).

The outcome is a vivid demonstration of the kind of alliance described by Cohen (1985), in which participants with quite different motives and interests find themselves advancing the same control policies. Over 'punishment in the community', the probation service, the government, penal reformers, and the public come together. Events in the last decade have demonstrated that rehabilitative approaches cannot be more expensive or less effective than 'short' – or long – 'sharp shocks'. The probation service also represents the humane response to offending which many support when faced with a real offender rather than offenders in the abstract. Police public relations is now focused on re-educating the public to see crime as a pervasive social fact not containable simply by police action (Chibnall 1977; Cohen 1985; Schlesinger *et al.* 1991).

During the 1980s the weakening of local government autonomy and the interpretation of media profile as a measure of quasi-market effectiveness in other parts of the public sector have undermined conventional elective democracy as the basis of legitimacy. It is, therefore, unlikely that the new world of image-building, corporate logos and competitive profiling will go away. It would seem that in this new arena of struggle the probation service is better placed than local authority social services. While it can no longer be thankful for being 'no news', it has the possibility of presenting its work as 'good news', in both the local and the national press. It is, though, competing not only with the rest of the state criminal justice industry, but with the voluntary sector. While finance may not be directly at stake, attention and approval are themselves a scarce resource. In these respects the voluntary sector has in-built advantages where the press is concerned, as we shall see in the next chapter.

Chapter 6

Good news about social work

Bad news about social work, far from spotlighting every seeming failure of every type of agency with every client group in every media outlet is, in reality, highly discriminating. Its epicentre is policy failures and practice errors in local authority social services. Even these are covered very selectively, only getting into the national press when the issue has aspects which tie to the wider news agendas of particular newspapers. For local papers the threshold of relevance is far lower, but the standing of the department as authoritative source accordingly higher.

What does good news about social work look like? 'No news' cannot be the answer for state social work, however attractive that might seem. As public agencies social services departments and the probation service must be available to scrutiny. To claim that this can be achieved solely by access to the public benches at committee meetings or through the electoral process, while formally correct, is now unrealistic. Technocracy and paternalism have been challenged by both right and left. Skill at self-promotion is now used as a criterion of fitness for purpose by right-wing advocates of competition and markets. The new reality is that all social work agencies must have media strategies, being ready to present a constructive response to things going badly and continuously to promote their activities when things are going well.

In considering how social work might be good news, it is useful to distinguish not only between media, and between agencies, but to consider the relevance of the work itself. This chapter will fall into three sections. Evidence about the potential (and risks) of local press coverage from previous chapters will be reviewed and expanded. The symbiotic relationship between voluntary organizations and the news media will be explored, using NACRO, the NSPCC and ChildLine as illustrations. There is, though, one aspect of local authority social services operations which is thought routinely to get a 'good press': griefwork in disasters. What are the extent and significance of this?

SUDDENLY SOCIAL WORK IS A GOOD THING

'It is now part of the journalist's brief always to contact social services following disasters', writes Walder (1991: 214), a journalist who was appointed PRO to Bradford Social Services in 1987. The department's policy of pro-active media relations had been influenced by the experience of the first of what turned out to be a succession of calamities resulting in the loss of many lives in the UK during the late 1980s, the Bradford football stadium fire of May 1985 in which fifty-six people died.

> We were not always popular within [social services], or even the town, for initiating so much coverage for social work . . . I'm convinced that our stance in Bradford . . . has made other social services departments more prepared to be pro-active following such tragic disasters.
>
> (Walder 1991: 213)

Much of Walder's very interesting discussion describes her practical efforts to make Bradford staff more media literate and confident. She does not, though, draw out the significant differences between news media. As we have seen, broadcasting works within statutory requirements to be 'impartial'. Her educative work with print journalists involved the local press, which can have only limited, indirect impact in taming the highly partial national press by influencing the framing of stories which may get picked up, or be passed on by stringers and news agencies. She does not reveal whether an attempt to contain a local 'child vice' story by providing tabloid-friendly case histories to national papers was judged successful. The profile of social services' work in disasters projected in the national press is similarly ambiguous.

After the *Herald of Free Enterprise* capsized off Zeebrugge in March 1987, with the loss of 193 lives, Kent Social Services set up a complex operation to counsel survivors and bereaved relatives throughout the UK. Establishing this 'outreach to a nation' (*Community Care* 15 September 1988) took several weeks and may well have figured in occasional news items during its work, which lasted until three weeks after the first anniversary of the disaster. Certainly, though, social work involvement did not feature in the news coverage of the disaster and its immediate aftermath. The only national daily papers to mention griefwork at all were the *Daily Telegraph* (8 March 1987) and *The Independent* (10 March 1987). The *Telegraph* used a psychiatrist as their expert voice on trauma, while *The Independent* quoted Colin Murray Parkes (very well known for his writing on bereavement and loss) and Cruse (originally a self-help group for widows, but now working more widely with bereavement). Social services had not yet become visible players or authorized knowers.

Nor had the situation changed by the first anniversary of the sinking. On 7 March 1988 *Today*, the *Sun*, the *Daily Mirror* and the *Daily Mail* covered the event (quite extensively in the latter two cases). Social services were not mentioned. There was nothing at all in the *Daily Telegraph* and *The Independent*.

By the end of that year, however, griefwork had become part of the repertoire of standard news angles. In December 1988 three morning commuter trains collided in an inner London suburb. Thirty-six people died and 111 were injured. The crash was given intensive coverage in the national daily papers: it was very accessible, very visual, fitted the daily schedule perfectly – and was all too understandable to the readership. The most extensive coverage was in *Today*, which allocated twelve pages to the accident.

The news coverage of the Clapham crash in a sample of national daily papers was scrutinized for the period from the day after (Tuesday, 13 December 1988) until the end of that week. All the papers sampled took up the issue of dealing with trauma. The contribution to the public standing of local authority social services work was, though, blunted by the predominant medicalization of the issue, noticeably in the right-wing papers. Only the *Guardian* (14 December 1988) was specific:

> Meanwhile, social services staff in Dorset, where one of the trains began its journey, have set up special telephone helplines. They offer assistance and counselling to families of the bereaved and injured drawing on experience from the Hungerford and King's Cross incidents [respectively a mass shooting by a deranged man and a fire on the London Underground].
>
> (*Guardian* 14 December 1988)

Even here, though, the attention given to social services is in the last paragraph of an article in which a psychiatrist was used to frame the issue.

Elsewhere, social work was consigned to a generalized and/or subordinate role. During the harrowing process of identifying personal possessions, 'In a next-door room [at the local police station] 15 Salvation Army officers and social workers sat, hearing the cries of grief and waiting in case there was anything they could offer to assuage such anguish' (*Daily Mirror* 14 December 1988). 'A team of social workers and counsellors are standing by to help the families of the victims' (*The Times* 13 December 1988). Two days later (15 December) a background article in *The Times* centred on the counselling available from a team 'led by' the consultant psychiatrist at the local hospital. His liaising with Wandsworth Social Services to set up a 'hotline' and the work of social workers on the wards were also mentioned.

The *Daily Express* coverage (13 December) also used a psychiatrist as expert on post-traumatic stress, while the extremely detailed coverage in *Today* merely made a passing mention of the Salvation Army. On 15 December, in a follow-up article, that paper gave a full column to the effect on hospital staff of treating victims: 'Psychiatrists, social workers and the hospital chaplain are helping the nurses . . .'.

Many such tragic events have a political dimension. At Clapham it emerged soon enough to feature in the immediate newspaper response. While the *Daily Mirror* was asking about the impact of public expenditure cuts on railway safety (14 December), the *Sun*'s two-deck headline on its double page spread ran 'WHO IS THE BRITISH RAIL BODGER?' (14 December), which serves as a reminder that it is not only hapless social workers who are pursued in the search for individual blame. Not that the *Sun* neglected the newly understood importance of the emotional injury caused by such terrible incidents, even if the style bordered on self-parody. Beside the 'bodger' headline is a single column on '10 WAYS TO BEAT GRIEF', with the headline in white-on-black and the '10' in a starburst. (The advice which follows is relevant and clearly expressed, presumably provided by Cruse, contact details of which appear at the end.)

Party politics were less visible in the search to explain the meaning and implications of the death by crushing of ninety-six people at the Hillsborough football stadium, Sheffield, in April 1989. The horrible events did, however, throw up fundamental questions about the institutional order, which inflected news coverage at the time and reverberate still. These centred on the appropriateness of police preparations and reaction, the behaviour of fans, and the underlying orientation of football as a profit-driven capitalist business to its consumers, historically treated as working-class turnstile fodder. In a memorable piece of London-centric ignorance and bad taste, the *Sun* fell back on its reflex individualism, accusing Liverpool supporters of drunken loutish behaviour and, by extension, attributing the events to crowd violence (see Chippindale and Horrie (1990) for further background). This whole interpretative framework has since been discredited; the *Sun* lost a considerable proportion of its sales on Merseyside and has never regained it. In contrast, on 20 April a *Today* leader was extremely critical of the police.

Association football is still the British national game; the occasion was a major cup match involving Liverpool, one of the most avidly supported of clubs. The whole nightmare took place in front of television cameras. It is, therefore, not surprising that all news media were dominated by Hillsborough for days after. On 17 April, for example, the *Daily Telegraph* gave it the whole of its first five pages, while the *Sun* filled sixteen pages. What follows is commentary on a sample of national daily papers for the first week after the tragedy.

As with the Clapham crash, the news treatment of the help offered to survivors and the bereaved shows a reluctance by the right-wing tabloids to attribute a lead responsibility to local authority social work, either in the construction of stories or in lexicalization. (It must be said, though, that of the papers sampled only the *Daily Mirror* failed to develop the griefwork dimension.) The 'expert' who provides advice in the *Sun* is a psychiatrist (17 April), although the Liverpool 'council' helpline is mentioned. On 21 April, according to the *Sun*, '150 cops need tragedy counselling'. Fittingly in an enterprise culture, private consultants are to be used.

Private enterprise was also to the fore in the *Daily Mail*, where the 'managing director of the Centre for Clinical Psychiatry' had been 'called to Liverpool to *teach* the social workers who are manning helplines'. In this account, the Director of Social Services is quoted and his department credited with '*co-ordinating* the counselling services' (*Daily Mail* 18 April 1988; my emphases).

This contrasts with the account in *The Independent* (22 April): 'Liverpool's Social Services director ... who is *in charge of* [my emphasis] a massive effort to counsel hundreds of people affected by the tragedy, said yesterday that more than 900 people had contacted his department for help.' The full-page background feature included a prominent picture of the department's 'disaster advice centre'.

The *Daily Telegraph* provided an intermediate representation of state social work. On 17 April 'teams of clergymen, social workers and psychiatrists' were 'comforting relatives of the dead'. Later on in the coverage the Director of Sheffield Social Services was quoted directly on his department's response and experience, drawn in part from colleagues elsewhere. On 19 April a further article described the counselling as being 'co-ordinated' by Liverpool Social Services, 'with the help of voluntary groups and churches'. Staff will also require 'special training from experts in crisis psychology'. The need for specialist advice in such exceptional circumstances is not surprising, but the stress on the 'outsideness' of the expertise tends to imply a lack of professional knowledge within the department and wider profession.

Four conclusions can be drawn from this case material. Three have already become evident. First, that seeking out the counsellors is now a standard newsgathering task when a 'disaster' occurs. Second, this does not necessarily mean extensive laudatory accounts of what social services do. As we have seen, some coverage is framed in terms of 'trying hard despite lack of expertise'. At best a senior figure may be given an opportunity to speak with authority in the context of a hard news-style account because, third, those newspapers whose politics cast social services as part of the 'dependency culture' do not abandon their stance.

The fourth dimension is implicit in the news treatment: this is social work for the deserving, the majority, tax-paying normals. 'People who have never used social workers before and hardly knew what they did', as it was put in a *Community Care* article (1 September 1988) about the work of the Grampian Social Work Department after the Piper Alpha oil rig explosion and fire. Being caught up in a disaster is, by definition, haphazard and implies no failure of individual responsibility. This is an unusual opportunity for social service work to reach a wider public, through both the griefwork itself and the news media discussion.

Social understandings of trauma, stress and their emotional consequences have changed profoundly. Television coverage of the 1991 Gulf War included front-line pilots talking about returning from missions and crying with relief. Firefighters broken by what happened to them at King's Cross have been compensated at a level once reserved for physical injury. Can this be attributed to the influence of social work? Realistically not: the more likely cause is the widespread penetration of popular psychology through manifold routes like the self-help movement, women's 'general-interest' magazines, the rapidly growing market for health magazines, and radio and television quasi-counselling shows. 'Let's talk about me', originating in the US, has taken hold easily given the deep roots of English individualism and the hegemony of English culture in the UK (Aldridge 1990). There is much that is positive about the valorization of the affective beside the cognitive and physical, but at its worst this view of the self and society is one in which mental health is commodified into a set of do-it-yourself tools, and blaming the patient for the illness is very near the surface. Systematic inequities are defined away. For this reason, the counselling expertise of social services departments as a vehicle for positive news management must be treated with profound caution. It has the potential to undermine policies and practice justified at the level of the social structure and distributive justice.

THE VIEW FROM THE LOCAL PAPER

When social workers say 'What would this look like in the papers?', the probability is that any publicity would appear in the local rather than the national press. Even here, social work does not figure as often as social workers' apprehension would suggest. During my monitoring of the Nottingham *Evening Post* during May, June and July 1991, there were fifty-eight days with no mention of social work (73 per cent of the total); one day when probation featured; three when specific voluntary agencies were covered; and fifteen when social services – the second biggest spending department in the county – were mentioned.

From a pragmatic point of view 'good news' must be understood to mean not just positive – even promotional – coverage, but neutral treatment, and the opportunity to respond in sufficient and accurately reported detail to bad news.

Yet even praise is possible. According to the Midlands probation officer handling media relations (see Chapter 5), local free papers respond better to stories with pictures of real people. The same imperative for personalization and identification is true of the paid-for press and can be used to drive effective 'good news'. On 20 July 1991, for example, the Nottingham *Evening Post* published a substantial feature on a 'pioneering project' run jointly by health and social services to support homeless people with mental health problems – not an obviously appealing group. The whole text is given to a sympathetic account of the extent and cause of their need for support, and is illustrated with pictures of two of the team members and of a local man whose death had provided part of the impetus for the project. As we have also seen from the work of the south-western probation service PRO in Chapter 5, local affiliation can make other apparently unlikely subjects, like the work of offenders on community service, victim support schemes, and probation staff promotions, into positive news.

The relatively infrequent references to social work in the *Evening Post* were not an aberration; by chance my sample period included the reopening of the major local issue 'Save Our Homes' (see Chapter 4) and three national controversies involving social work. Nevertheless, most of the reports were framed as hard news in neutral for-and-against format. Where an issue attracted editorial comment a valiant effort not to over-simplify was often evident. On occasion this produced equivocation worthy of the *Guardian* itself!

At the end of May and beginning of June 1991 the *Evening Post* had a succession of stories on the problems of 'how best to protect children in care' (*EP* 7 June 1991). On 29 and 31 May two brief articles summarized the implications of the pin-down inquiry report (Levy and Kahan 1991). The local salience was highlighted by a p. 1 item (31 May) reporting that Nottinghamshire Social Services was reviewing the lessons to be learned. This was linked presentationally and in a leader comment to the p. 1 lead '"CARE GIRLS" SEX TRADE SHOCK'. Despite the lurid headline, the theme of the text is that police, social services and magistrates are working together on a difficult dilemma. As the editorial comment says: 'are the staff to keep the youngsters locked up day after day in the manner of the "pindown" homes or are they to give them a reasonable amount of freedom to "rehabilitate" them in a relaxed atmosphere?' (Nottingham *Evening Post* 31 May 1991). The conclusion is inescapably along the lines that 'something must be done' – but the tone is sympathetic to the social work task. A similar lack of narrative closure was evident in a full-page feature on the same topic in the paper on 7 June, and another on 'Crime kiddies' the following day.

Local residents must figure well up a local paper's hierarchy of credibility. They are described as 'understandably angry' at disturbance from a local children's home in another *Evening Post* leader on 2 June 1991, and then congratulated for not demanding its closure. This time the paper is critical of social services, but of management's failure to act rather than of its rationale or front-line staff. Indeed, the care workers are defended: 'It's the age-old difficulty . . . of staff on low wages who are not experienced enough to handle the rowdies . . . browbeating them with threats of closure doesn't seem to be an adequate or sensible quick fix to the problem.'

Another vivid illustration of the sensitive relationship between a local paper and its readership also occurred during my sample period. A very senior member of social services was disciplined for expressing religiously motivated personal views, with implications for the work of the department, in a television debate. The unions strongly objected; there were public demonstrations and petitions in his support; the issue was raised in parliament; it made the national news and several articles in the social work trade press. The *Evening Post* gave the controversy detailed coverage, but made no leader comment.

During a trial the news treatment must be neutral (not that this protects against the reporting of accusations by the judge or counsel). When social work really does become 'bad news' the sheer volume of local press coverage must itself be a source of pressure on the staff of the department concerned. We have already seen examples of saturation coverage in the Charlene Salt case (in Chapter 2) and the Frank Beck trial (in Chapter 3).

Whatever the tone of the coverage, the sense of bombardment can only be increased where several local papers serve the same or overlapping areas, perhaps an evening paper, weekly paid-fors and weekly free papers. Apart from common sources and simple borrowing of material, the absorption of many free papers into the same corporate ownership as the paid-fors (see Franklin and Murphy 1991) suggests that the same interpretative framework may well appear several times.

In most cases the volume of coverage may be offset by all those forces which incline local papers to a less partisan style, as we saw with the *Leicester Mercury* and Frank Beck, and the Nottingham *Evening Post* in its return to a more conciliatory line over the elderly persons' home saga. On occasion, though, other aspects of the news agenda will put pressure on staff and departments. Although the Oldham *Evening Chronicle* did not mount a concerted attack on the social services over the Charlene Salt case, the paper's tabloid popular news format, with its emphasis on pictured and named persons, resulted in a focus on the senior social worker involved.

On occasion the local press, like the national press, will anyway be predisposed to a particular explanatory paradigm. In the summer of 1992 her mother and her mother's partner were jailed for the manslaughter of 4-year-old Sophie Merry at Lewes Crown Court. (Both subsequently appealed.) The evidence revealed a gruesome history of violence and squalor; the accused were well known to statutory agencies. Police and probation, as well as social services, had carried out internal inquiries, all of which were alluded to in local press coverage. Nevertheless, the Brighton *Evening Argus* focused its leader comments almost entirely on the blameworthiness of social services, laying heavy emphasis on parallels with the Maria Colwell case nineteen years before. In that case the same paper had mounted a high-profile campaign (see Chapter 7).

Quite apart from the commercial risks in local papers vilifying all and sundry, the very extent of local coverage of social work 'disasters' has constructive aspects. There will be space for a detailed account, not only of 'what went wrong' but the inevitably complex circumstances, and what steps have been or will be taken to rectify the situation. A major arm of local government is bound to be treated as authoritative by the local press. If the response is informative, coherent and not fragmented by internal conflict, much can be achieved. There can be few instance of 'bad news' in social work worse than the Frank Beck case. Yet the revelations of breathtaking complacency and inaction in the *Leicester Mercury*'s lengthy extracts from the Newell report provide a paradoxical sense of reassurance: they serve as signs of the seriousness and effectiveness of the remedial action. More space offers the possibility of more under-standing; less space usually means more simplification; simplification often means personalized blame.

This is very bad news indeed for state social work in London, where the daily evening paper has a mass readership analogous to a national daily. It can afford to be accordingly partial – its news pitch is right-wing mid-market with quasi-broadsheet features. Local papers in London are enfeebled by less stable and distinctive area-based identification. Neither social services nor probation can benefit from the direct cultivation of good relationships and the market-driven editorial prudence which offer possibilities to provincial agencies.

Despite the possibilities of constructive contact with the local press (and broadcasting), there is no doubt that local authority social services face manifold difficulties in media relations. Their responsibilities are multiplex; success is often hard to demonstrate; relations between paid staff and elected members are always delicate – and much of the national press wants welfare services contained. (The problems of social work's mission are discussed in more detail in Chapters 7 and 8.) Conversely, media coverage is crucial to the existence of many voluntary agencies. Their strategies and the treatment they receive make an instructive comparison.

SELLING SOCIAL WORK – THE VOLUNTARY SECTOR

'Conservative governments of the 1980s saw the voluntary sector as innovative, flexible, participatory, potentially cost-effective but, above all, as independent of the State' (Waine 1992: 84). Whatever the realities of their philosophy, effectiveness, or actual source of funding, voluntary organizations could be made to represent all the virtues of decentral-ization, individual decision, responsiveness to the consumer, and entrepreneurial-style self-help. Better still, they were a ready-made vehicle for the development of welfare pluralism by acting as providers to health services and local authorities. In fact many voluntary organiza-tions, far from being supported by corporate sponsorship or the successful rattling of collecting tins, receive large amounts of state funds. Schlesinger *et al.* (1991) report that in 1989–90 the National Association for Victim Support Schemes was receiving £4 million from the Home Office, for example.

Putting this political favour together with the dependence of many voluntary organizations upon publicity for both their campaigning goals and their fund-raising immediately suggests that their relationship with

the news media, particularly the national press, will be very different from
that of state social work. To explore this contrast further, I selected three
voluntary organizations. NACRO works in the area of criminal justice,
the NSPCC with children and families, and ChildLine with children.

NACRO is a well-established voluntary organization with its
headquarters in London, and a strong network of local branches. Its work
in support of offenders and ex-offenders has two tracks. One is acting as
a pressure group instigating and reacting to criminal justice policy and
practice: it is a major player in this 'policy community' (Schlesinger *et
al.* 1991, quoting Kingdon 1984). NACRO also does direct work like
running bail hostels, post-release accommodation and employment
schemes. As much of its funding comes through central government for
these projects, money does not have to be solicited from the public at
large. It can, therefore, afford to diverge from popular beliefs about crime
and criminals. In the view of NACRO, the attitude of the public (and of
offenders) to offending is punitive, but this does not seem to affect the
work or standing of the organization – even when clients go awry.
Presumably it shares with the probation service a clear position on 'our'
side of the deviance boundary, with some additional licence for restrained
radicalism conferred by its voluntary status.

NACRO has a tight, centrally directed policy on media relations. A
NACRO Procedures leaflet on dealing with the news media contains
detailed advice. Local branches are encouraged to seek local publicity for
their work (and seem to succeed – see below) but all comment on matters
of penal policy must come from senior headquarters staff, where a
specific group deals with press and broadcast media approaches for
background material and reaction/comment. The organization has a
strong line on 'damage limitation': branches are directed to seek
immediate guidance from the centre in dealing with bad publicity.
Criticism always gets a response, in the form of counter-facts, which,
according to NACRO, tend to be reported if they come from the director.
Letters to the newspapers are systematically written and considered a
powerful tool, being 'among the most widely read parts of . . . papers'
(*NACRO Procedures no. 2* 1990).

In its pro-active work, NACRO is addressing the broadsheet and local
press and the broadcast media. The mass tabloids are not targeted,
because of both lack of take-up (which corresponds with NAPO's
experience reported in Chapter 5 and is confirmed by my sample of
NACRO's cuttings) and the explicit orientation of some, in particular the
Sun, to sex offenders and homosexuality.

The organization has the advantage of a clear set of objectives and can

often produce very concrete 'news', although the demand for personalization by focusing on real participants in its schemes can present a
problem. 'If the offender is articulate, willing and fully aware of the
possible drawbacks, this can be a useful way of making the message more
vivid for the listener, viewer or reader' (*NACRO Procedures no. 2* 1990).
However, the guidance goes on to counsel project members on the
possible pitfalls; some staff are uneasy about asking offenders to respond
to news media requests at all.

NACRO is clearly treated with respect by the press, even when in
critical mode. The organization's response to the government's electronic
tagging proposals was extremely hostile (as was NAPO's – see Chapter
5), but was reported without adverse comment in three national daily
papers (*The Times*, the *Daily Telegraph* and the *Financial Times*), four
regional dailies and nine further local papers – as well as the *Sunday
Times* and the women's magazine *Chat*. (NACRO routinely circulates
women's magazines, but does not produce material specifically aimed at
this sector.)

In June 1991 NACRO issued ten news releases, three of which were
on very local matters. Four of the remainder got a significant response. A
release on the high number of 'lifers' in the UK was used by the *Mail on
Sunday*, the *Friend* – the magazine of the Religious Society of Friends
(Quakers) – and eleven regional/local papers. Material on the 'league
table' of the UK's most overcrowded prisons, was used by three national
broadsheets, the *Mail on Sunday* and thirty local papers. Many of these
added further material relating to prisons in their readership area. The
same pattern of response followed a release on the UK's having
proportionately the highest prison population in Europe, with mentions in
three national broadsheets, two national mid-market tabloids, one
regional paper, and twenty-one local papers, a few of which elaborated
on the NACRO material. Only *The Times* and three local papers took up
NACRO's response to a Home Office announcement on policy on sex
offenders.

NACRO's clippings collection for the same period contained
twenty-five clippings of unsolicited news, six from national and nineteen
from local media. Four of the national references were using NACRO as
'authorized knower'. Only one of the whole twenty-five could be
described as adverse: a policemen in St Albans attacking organizations
like NACRO for lobbying magistrates for 'leniency' – to which a reply
had been sent. Even 'bad news' of failed schemes and a scheme member
in court was covered in neutral terms. Eleven local items were actual
'good news', based on staged events set up by local branches. Some of

the take-up was by free papers, underlining their potential if the right formula is applied.

In direct contrast to NACRO, in 1991 only 7 per cent of the funding of the NSPCC (the National Society for the Prevention of Cruelty to Children) came from local and central government, while 86 per cent originated from legacies and 'raised voluntary income' (*NSPCC Background Notes* 1992). Since this proportion amounted to over £27 million, the society must address the public in as many ways as possible. This can result in contradictions and curious juxtapositions, as we shall see.

The society, founded in Liverpool in 1884, is deeply embedded in British life in both a popular and a structural sense. For many years it operated through uniformed inspectors – the 'cruelty man'. The post-war expansion of state social work inevitably raised questions about the continuing need for the NSPCC, but an accommodation was reached with local authority social services. Occasional outbreaks of conflict over policy and practice still occur, however (Parton 1985; 1991). The unique institutional place of the society is manifested in two ways. It is legally established, remaining the only non-statutory body with 'authorized person' status under successive child protection legislation, i.e. 'the right to remove children from the home without the police but with the consent of a Justice of the Peace' (NSPCC 1992: 5). The NSPCC is also part of the social establishment, enjoying the active patronage of royalty. HRH the Princess Margaret is president; one-third of the 1991 executive committee were titled. Entertainment industry celebrities often work on its behalf.

Uniforms were finally abandoned in 1969; Child Protection Officers now work within a network of local Child Protection Teams. Decision-making on both direct work and local fund-raising is increasingly being decentralized to the regions. National media relations are, though, co-ordinated centrally by a staff of four within the headquarters communications group, which produces materials and deals with the advertising for the society's campaigns and national fund-raising events.

Contact with the news media is 50:50 reactive to pro-active. Both national and local news organizations use the NSPCC as a source not only of comment but of unattributed background information for news and features. Providing answers to queries like 'What is the minimum age for a babysitter?' is considered well worth the investment of resources because of the good relations that are built up. When news involving the welfare of children breaks, the society finds that it is always approached. If local, the matter will be referred to regional organizations (and usually the relevant social services department as well). Major issues like new legislation or national controversies will probably result in calls to comment or to give interviews from high-status broadcast media programmes, for example the BBC Radio 4 *Today* programme and the BBC *Nine O'Clock News*, as well as from the national press. The society attributes this constant request to be the expert voice to its high profile; to being national in scope and non-political; to its expertise; and to its reliability and responsiveness.

In its pro-active media work, the NSPCC's main aims are twofold. It tries to educate about the problems with which it deals while stressing its accessibility. Second, it needs to raise very large sums of money.

As social conditions change, any voluntary organization must adapt or disappear. The NSPCC has inevitably, as a third strand of activity, played an active part in the very definition of social problems. Parton (1985: 58ff.) describes the organization's central role in the naming of the battered child syndrome. It set up a special unit in 1968, coinciding with its renegotiated relationship to expanding state social work. During the 1980s it was pivotal in developing paradigms of aetiology and practice in child sexual abuse. This was the subject of a major campaign in 1985 (Soothill and Walby 1991: 113ff.); workers at the Rochdale NSPCC unit were particularly influential (Parton and Parton 1989). So attracting news media interest is vital to the pursuit of this aim too, but not all NSPCC campaigning and educational work is media-based. Direct contact is made with MPs and professionals through briefings, conferences and seminars. A university-based researcher is funded. Open days are held at local projects.

Given its mission and present scale of activities, though, the public has to be the NSPCC's main target. High-profile campaigns are run on an annual cycle, with a news release, a launching press conference, an elaborate media pack, an advertising campaign and leaflets in versions designed for specific audiences (for instance, for young people on the meaning of child abuse; for teachers on identifying and responding to it; for the public to explain what happens if they report their suspicions). The publication of the annual report is also used to make an impact in the news media.

The extent of media exposure is monitored closely. Clippings from the national newspapers (tabloids as well as broadsheets), the social work trade press and women's magazines are collected at headquarters, which also gets reports of national and local broadcast media coverage through its subscription to an agency. Local print media reaction is also monitored through an agency and forwarded to the regions. According to headquarters staff, 'Most of the 800 local papers mention the NSPCC at least once a month'.

The NSPCC autumn campaign in 1991, 'Act Now for Children', used as its springboard research findings showing widespread uncertainty about how to identify and respond to child abuse. Launch day was 26 September. On 27 September 1991, according to NSPCC clippings files, items appeared in the *Guardian*, the *Daily Telegraph*, *Today*, the *Daily Star*, the *Sun*, and the *Daily Mirror* (as well as in regional/local papers, the London *Evening Standard*, the Salvation Army *War Cry*, the *Christian Herald*, the *Caribbean Times* and the *Asian Times*). The format of the news treatment was predictably varied. The broadsheets described the aims of the launch in brief bylined articles without illustration, clearly based on the news release. In the mass tabloids, coverage centred on photo-opportunities of women 'showbiz stars' (*Daily Star* 27 September 1991) holding 'one-year-old Alex' (*Sun* 27 September 1991), who looked photogenic but a bit apprehensive, on their shoulders. Both the *Sun* and the *Daily Mirror* allocated three sentences of text to the story – but 25 column cm and 30 column cm respectively to the picture. Only the *Daily Star* described the aims of the campaign.

For *Today* the launch was part of a continuing story which had started with an 'exclusive' on 16 September 1991: 'CHILDREN IN NEW DANGER; Orkneys backlash puts thousands more at risk'. The p. 1 lead was followed by extensive coverage, with pictures, and leader comment on pp. 4 and 5, based on a 'dramatic report . . . compiled by *Today* in association with the NSPCC and Scotland Yard'. The message of the text is that news media attention to the events in Cleveland, Rochdale and Orkney has confused the public. According to the editorial 'Many people now believe that this kind of abuse does not really happen . . . caring neighbours are reluctant to report their suspicion because they think they could instigate an unnecessary family break-up'. The writer goes on to affirm that the child should be seen 'as an individual who has rights' and that we must 'learn to trust the experts', because abuse, including sexual abuse, is very real.

The official launch of the campaign was given prominent treatment in *Today*, and on 2 October 1991 there was more: a double page spread on 'Loving care that led a child in torment to pour out her secret in drawing', describing in detail a case study of the work of a child protection officer.

Today's intensive coverage of the campaign is in marked contrast to the other mid-market tabloids, the *Daily Mail* and the *Daily Express*, which appear not to have reported it. This is consistent with their pro-traditional family market niche, which may in itself explain *Today*'s commitment. During the period in question the paper was trying to establish itself as the only non-Tory national paper in the Murdoch stable, pitched at younger white-collar family-orientated readers. Human interest material with an informative and mildly progressive content would obviously fit very well with this agenda, especially if much of the background research was ready-made. The byline 'Education Correspondent' on the 2 October feature appears to confirm *Today*'s stretched editorial resources, much commented upon in the newspaper trade press.

News releases from the NSPCC are not only linked to high-visibility campaigns and events. During the period May to July 1992, headquarters issued sixteen. Five were on policy issues, including: the risks to children in residential care; the legal status of physical punishment; the launch of a joint educational initiative with the Family Rights Group; and comments on the Child Support Act, which seeks to extract financial support from absent fathers. Both this and the release calling for the outlawing of physical punishment were critical of government policy and implicit attitudes. The stance on punishment produced the only national press mention of the NSPCC during the sample period which could be construed as hostile. The *Daily Express* (4 May 1992; also see Chapter 1) called in aid right-thinking people like Sir Nicholas Fairbairn and Dame Jill Knight MP to balance the views of the Scottish Law Commission, psychologists and voluntary groups, including the NSPCC. Although the format was standard for-and-against, the paper's agenda is clear: 'there are fears that the courts could be filled with families at war … Even Royal Family members could be on the wrong end of the law'.

The other eleven news releases during the study period related to media-geared fund-raising ranging from the collection of old-style 5p pieces, through several sporting events, to a 'Royal Charity Gala' attended by Princess Margaret, Norma Major (wife of the Prime Minister) and Terry Wogan (a very well-known television chat-show host). There was also pre-publicity for a concert and dinner to mark the 1992 autumn campaign, the patron of which was to be the Lord Chancellor, England's most senior law officer. Most of the other releases also gave at least a couple of weeks' advance notice, providing media with all-important predictable news (see Chapter 1).

Sifting the clippings of national press items for the May to July 1992 period showed, apart from the *Express* piece already described, the *Daily Mail* and the *Sun* using the NSPCC for expert comment, in the latter case on the wisdom of holding a 'Miss Wet T-shirt' contest for 5-year-olds (29 June). *Today*, the *Daily Express* and the *Daily Star* covered a fashion show in aid of the NSPCC – although the latter two did not name the cause. On both 5 May and 8 May the *Sun* devoted a whole page to a parachute jump, sponsored by the paper for the NSPCC, 'which does marvellous work to help children in need'. There were also mentions in the London *Evening Standard*, the *Sunday Times*, *Cycling Weekly*, and *Hello!* – twice.

Unlike those pressure groups whose dialogue is with the 'policy community', the NSPCC must seek whatever publicity it can. National broadcast media are found to be responsive, if the need for 'visuals' is met, as are local broadcasters to local campaigns (and some national issues – the 'smacking' news release was taken up by nine local radio stations). In general national press coverage, when it occurs, is favourable. Common ground must be found with the mass tabloids. They are vital for the NSPCC, not only because of the sheer size of their audience, but because the high proportion of their readers in the population must mean that many people needing help can be reached through their pages. In fact popular papers are seen as responding better to charities and will run campaigns themselves, unlike the broadsheets. If the format is right – personalization for social issues, celebrity photocalls for fundraising – the NSPCC has found that the mass tabloids report their initiatives accurately even if briefly, as we have seen.

NSPCC/news media relations seem to function well but this should not be confused with the absence of complexity. The society's work involves the secret recesses of family life, using professional skills that are constantly questioned. It needs support from every stratum of society and from media of all political hues. Ambiguities abound; consider two examples.

First, here is an organization the list of whose patrons, honorary officers, committee members and sponsors reads like a directory of the UK 'great and good'. Many will have attended public (that is, private) schools and will send their children there. Only recently has the extent of sanctioned physical punishment and unsanctioned sexual and physical abuse in such schools been acknowledged and questioned. Yet the NSPCC is making statements supporting the banning of physical punishment. How far could it develop this stance?

Second, during the summer of 1992 details of a phone conversation between the Princess of Wales and a close male friend were published and subsequently could be heard by calling a *Sun* phone line. The paper, criticized for not only publishing but profiting from this breach of privacy, offered the revenue (estimated at £50,000) to the NSPCC. The society refused it, despite the importance of the *Sun*'s huge readership – and a £2 million funding deficit.

We have seen that most news media organizations are actively well disposed to the NSPCC. The broadsheets respond to its professional pronouncements; its dramatic work with 'innocents' is a tabloid dream of reader identification, titillation and sentimentality – however careful the society is in framing it. Mid- and mass-market tabloids also make full use of its events in their symbiotic relationship with celebrities and royalty. The voluntary sector is favoured by the political right and left, so the politics of particular newspapers is unusually irrelevant. What happens when this comfortable relationship is threatened? The NSPCC was at the centre of the Rochdale débâcle and the RSPCC (its Scottish equivalent) played a lead role in the Orkney events. In the case of Rochdale (see Chapter 3), for most newspapers the contradiction was easily solved: the NSPCC was either mentioned only in passing or completely ignored. In the Tracy Wilkinson case too (Chapter 2) the *Daily Mail*, the only paper to give the story major play, minimized NSPCC practice failures. Tonkin (*Community Care* 5 March 1987) demonstrates how media coverage of the Heidi Koseda case transformed bad practice by a member of the NSPCC staff into evidence of the society's effectiveness despite the scale of its task. This was facilitated by the NSPCC's itself using 'bad apple' imagery, symmetrical with the tabloids' own epistemology of social problems.

Media news values and routines also serve the society well in a less obvious way. We have seen the NSPCC's efforts to refocus public attention on the pervasiveness of physical abuse, accompanied by a shift in emphasis to the social factors which cause stress and precipitate violent behaviour. This is the edge of dangerous ground. Not only must the NSPCC remain non-political because of its charitable status, but to make the link between poverty, unemployment and systematic inequality, or between sexual abuse and gender relations, would be a fundamental challenge to the institutional order into which the charity is so firmly inserted.

Inevitably, therefore, the NSPCC presents its work in terms of alleviating symptoms and restoring family function. It has been very involved in the developing vocabulary of 'dangerousness' (Parton 1985; 1991; Parton and Parton 1989) with all its connotations of the identifiable and containable minority (probably working-class) and unchallenged majority (mostly white middle-class). This suits the imperatives of most media organizations very well: the mass tabloids (and many broadcast outlets) are uninterested in abstraction, side-lining even limited attempts at causal explanation, as Soothill and Walby's (1991: 113) account of the 1985 campaign illustrates. The mid-market papers are pro-patriarchal family. Even the broadsheets have tended to accept the NSPCC's interpretative frameworks (Parton 1985; Parton and Parton 1989).

The origins of ChildLine are as modern as the NSPCC's are historic. Arising out of unmet need identified through a television programme, it was set up in 1986 to provide a 24-hour free telephone counselling service for 'children in Britain in trouble or danger' (ChildLine 1992). Its base is in London; there are (at late 1992) four regional offices. Being directly in touch only with children and aiming to deal with problems as defined by its users make it unusual among children's charities. This by itself is the source of some adverse media comment, not so much through news treatment as by right-wing male columnists who take the view that its work exaggerates the scale of child abuse and encourages children to make false and malicious accusations. ChildLine's formal response to this is that such responses are only to be expected as it is working in a sensitive and controversial area.

Although ChildLine, like the NSPCC, has attracted extensive corporate sponsorship, and entertainment and other celebrities work on its behalf, its social base is more professional than establishment, with an advisory council drawn from state and voluntary social work.

The Director of Press and Public Relations works with three colleagues and support staff in the London office. As well as handling media relations, they produce the annual report, a newsletter, leaflets, posters and other campaign materials. Esther Rantzen, ChildLine's chair and original driving force, has a background in television journalism. Its executive director, Valerie Howarth, was director of social services in Brent at the time of the Jasmine Beckford case. Media policy is, accordingly, tight and centralized with a limited number of people authorized to represent the organization (Howarth 1991). Care is taken to speak with one voice, to keep internal dissent private – and to resist the temptation to comment on children's issues in general. As a result, after what it describes as 'initial hysteria', the organization has settled down to being a routine source of background information for a wide range of news media. 'Bad news' requiring damage limitation has been rare, usually centred on problems with staff or fund-raisers gone wrong.

In its pro-active mode, the organization is trying to reach as many people as possible. It sees itself as having a semi-educational task, besides communicating its availability to children. Raising money is also high priority. The charity continues to try to expand as calls are still going unanswered. Additional credibility with professionals and policy/political influentials is a welcome secondary effect of media coverage.

Media are targeted through news releases, news conferences, celebrity events, and calls to individual journalists. Any coverage in a national newspaper or broadcast media is prized. Hardest to achieve are mentions in the broadsheet dailies: they need to be actively persuaded of the relevance of the issue in question. The mass tabloids may also take an interest; the greatest resistance comes from the mid-market press, where the *Daily Mail* has been known to make use of publicity material without acknowledging ChildLine's part in the event. Coverage in the regional/local press is much easier to achieve because of its different news values and thresholds of attention, but is axiomatically more limited in potential impact.

More than most voluntary agencies, the communications media infuse ChildLine. It could even be described as a creature of the electronic media themselves, gestated, born and now nurtured by popular actuality coverage. There could be no ambivalence in the organization about working on media relations. Surely we should expect news media to be unusually well disposed to ChildLine? The reality is less simple.

As far as the national press is concerned, ChildLine starts with many of the advantages of the voluntary sector, including lack of party-political-based hostility, clarity of purpose, sophisticated media relations policies and resources – and it works with children. Nevertheless, the news media treatment of ChildLine, as with other voluntary agencies and state social work, depends upon the politics, editorial policies, news values, assets and routines of the media. While its mistakes are unlikely to be big news, favourable reporting is not guaranteed. For an organization dependent upon fund-raising, no news is undoubtedly bad news.

Comparing ChildLine with NACRO and the NSPCC also emphasizes that the relationship between charity, client group and the response of the commercial press is intricate. Working with offenders does not necessarily contaminate; working with children may be questioned if their rights are put too much in the foreground; being very large and well established may bring its own limitations in working for those you are trying to help. These considerations, of client confidentiality, public accountability, the right compromise between principles and public profile, good professional practice, political sensitivities and priorities in use of resources are actually much the same as those brandished by social services staff saying that they cannot treat with the media. Deconstructing the relationship between agency, client group and type of news media organization reveals that the voluntary sector is not the beneficiary of automatically accessed uncritical media coverage. Nor are local authority social services always and everywhere being attacked. The experience of voluntary organizations in their essential work with news media, taken together with those aspects of their responsibilities and the media outlets that provide social services with a 'good press', suggests many ways in which state social work could improve public understanding of its functions and be more effective when damage limitation is required.

Part III

Social work news and society

Chapter 7

Reacting to attack

Social work's preoccupation with its media coverage began after the death of Maria Colwell in 1973, the trial and conviction for manslaughter of her stepfather, and the subsequent public inquiry. This marked the transition of child abuse (initially called the 'battered baby syndrome' – see Parton (1985) for a comprehensive account) from the discourse of academic debate to that of social problem. The case made such an impact that, after twenty years and despite all the intervening controversies, 'another Colwell' is still used to call up the whole 'inventory' (Cohen 1973 and see Chapter 1) of intensive media scrutiny.

In 1978, Parsloe and Stevenson's authoritative research on daily practice in local authority social services commented on workers' anxiety about adverse media coverage (DHSS 1978: 320ff.). From the late 1970s social work's two weekly trade journals included articles about media coverage regularly enough to be an identified strand: 'Media Watch' in *Social Work Today*; 'The media' in *Community Care*. Concern reached its height during the mid-1980s when three highly publicized cases of murders of children in care occurred: Jasmine Beckford, Tyra Henry, Kimberley Carlile. The Association of Directors of Social Services set up a working party to consider the 'negative publicity' often attracted by social work (*Community Care* 13 March 1986). Since then there has been a decline in the journal space given to examining media coverage, even in respect of the Cleveland events of 1988, of which much has been written but little of it in social work journals. Between June 1991 and July 1992 there were no articles at all on the news media in *Social Work Today*, then the voice of the British Association of Social Workers. Yet the profession continues to be in the news over ritual child abuse and the widespread corruption of power to abuse children in residential care. These have been extensively covered in the trade press, but with little comment about media portrayal.

SOCIAL WORKERS REFLECT ON THEIR PRESS

Articles by practitioners in the social work press deal with two themes: what it is like to be the subject of media attention, and how the profession should react, both by supporting individuals and by setting up better professional and public relations mechanisms. It is important to note that, although the writers rarely specify, nearly all the discussion centres not on 'social work' but on local authority social services. Comment is rarely made on the very different experience of the probation service and of the big voluntary agencies carrying out direct work.

Reading the articles, three themes recur: personal pain; bewilderment; and a poor grasp of the functioning of the news media, either as daily work for its employees or as formal organizations occupying a key location in the social and political fabric. This last is ironic, given that many of the articles plead for more empathetic understanding of social work by newsgatherers.

Being the subject of unsolicited media attention can undoubtedly be a very unpleasant experience. The mass tabloids themselves call the intensive search for background material 'monstering'. (See Chippindale and Horrie (1990) for the *Sun* at work; Hollingsworth (1985) on the improper vilification of Labour candidate Peter Tatchell; Cm 1102 (1990) for the improper hounding of the popular television actor Gordon Kaye when he was seriously ill.) I will argue, however, that the pain and bewilderment expressed by social workers about adverse media treatment is made more acute by the philosophy and disputed knowledge base of the profession.

In 1979 *Social Work Today* ran an 'exclusive series' under the rather unfortunate title 'Tragedies revisited'. The first, on the Maria Colwell case (*Social Work Today* 9 January 1979), consists of two linked articles: a history of the case and its impact on the social services personnel involved, and a first-person account by the social worker who became the focus of the 'search for blame', Diana Lees. Interestingly Lees, who is reported in the article as needing protection as she came and went from the inquiry, says little about news media coverage as a source of personal distress. She reflects on her regret about Maria Colwell, her doubts about the value of inquiries, and her gratitude for the support of friends and colleagues. She is sometimes represented as having been driven out of social work by the Colwell controversy, but in her account the toll it took and the shaking of her confidence in her own professional judgement simply brought forward a decision to have a rest from practice eighteen months later, during which time she had become a team leader. Having done so, the pressures she had experienced made her reluctant to return.

'It had always seemed to me that no-one could go on being a social worker for years on end without a break to recharge the batteries . . . sometimes it was an effort to care, and this was quite distressing.'

In the background article, the social services director talks of the 'unfairness of public expectations and the way a very self-critical profession which needs comfort and support when things go wrong gets the reverse'. The symbolic power of the case is illustrated by a 1978 quotation from the Brighton *Evening Argus* 'MARIA WITNESS DIES IN HOSPITAL', about which the author, Ann Shearer, comments 'The story did nothing to lighten the grief of some of the people in headquarters that day'. (The witness referred to had been area director at the time.) The main thrust of the feature is the enormous impact that the Colwell trial and inquiry had on individuals, practice and formal procedures. Apart from the remark above, there is no criticism of media coverage. It is, rather, taken as a barometer of public concern: '*The Times* alone gave [the inquiry] 320 paragraphs', while the *Argus* gave the case 'saturation coverage'. The local paper is also credited with having been instrumental in the calling of a public rather than a local inquiry. Nevertheless there is an implicit assumption that the volume of media coverage whipped up public feeling and raised the temperature of the inquiry and its aftermath.

By 1983 the role of the media is being more clearly targeted as a problem. 'Social Worker 2 in the Lucie Gates case describes what it is like to be at the centre of Press interest in a child abuse inquiry' (*Community Care* 13 January 1983). The article is illustrated by a cartoon, about two-thirds the size of the text itself, of a journalist as a slavering dangerous dog – a curious choice for a journal, itself part of a large publishing conglomerate which then owned the *Daily Mirror*, addressing a profession so determined to drive out stereotyping. It opens, 'In recent years the national Press has consistently attacked and criticised social work. . . when a child falls though the welfare net society makes clear its disapproval through the media'. 'Social Worker 2' goes on to complain of the effect of publicity on other members of the family and the failure of management and of BASW to protect staff. S/he gives examples of dramatization and simplification in coverage and concludes with a call for better public relations work by BASW declaring 'Social workers need protection. They have personal needs . . . The press has to take responsibility for its role in social work functioning'.

Harbert (*Social Services Insight* 1–8 February 1986) also expects higher standards of responsibility from the press: 'Concepts of justice and civil liberties were totally ignored in the media comment' about the death of an elderly woman from hypothermia. The first quarter of his account is taken up with the obtuseness of local media in refusing to accept his initial reaction of 'no comment'.

A *Community Care* article (16 July 1987), this time under the tag 'Violence', also demonstrates resentment at newspapers' ability to impose an irrelevant or trivial interpretative framework on events. The author, Andrew Papworth, had been detained and threatened with a crossbow by a client. The mass tabloid accounts of the trial treated the episode as a joke: 'Giggles tie up court'. For Papworth, 'There *were* humorous aspects to it all but it was my prerogative to mention these when talking about these to friends and colleagues' (his emphasis).

One of the most extended accounts of media attention is by Martin Ruddock (1991), who was the 'receptacle for public anger' in the Kimberley Carlile trial and inquiry, the coverage of which is also described by Gaffaney (*Community Care* 28 May 1987). Ruddock vividly recounts the practicalities of being targeted by the news media: the shouted questions; being faced by banks of photographers; being asked to repeat his walk into the inquiry for the benefit of television news; endless phone calls to his family home; reporters camped outside; the fear that his family was being endangered; the need to get away and yet finding that the solitude of the North Yorkshire moors was no help – even 'the weather, sadly, seemed hostile and unfriendly' (Ruddock 1991: 109). At the end of the trial the *Daily Star* in particular gave it the 'monster' treatment that mass tabloids often devote to sensational court cases with a seven-page feature: '"Kim: It was Murder". Underneath this headline were three pictures: Nigel Hall's with the words "he killed her"; my picture with the words "he let her die" and finally Pauline Carlile's with "she betrayed her baby"' (Ruddock 1991: 110). Ruddock continues that the 'vitriol and anger' in the *Daily Star* and 'other papers' (he mentions the *Daily Mail* and the *Sun*) meant that it 'hurt to read it' particularly because it 'fed my own self-punishing feelings' (Ruddock 1991: 110).

Later on in the chapter, however, Ruddock draws attention to the ways in which he received sympathetic reporting. Having engaged a solicitor familiar with the mechanics of public controversy, he went on to the offensive and then detected a general improvement in media accounts. Specifically, he mentions the 'independent television production *Dispatches*', a *Guardian* article with extracts from his inquiry evidence, and Thames Television's *London Programme*, 'although a long interview was cut down merely to me communicating personal sadness at Kimberley's death' (Ruddock 1991: 114). The chapter concludes with five observations. The first is that 'the press crucified me but also gave me the means to communicate the reason why I believed the crisis had

occurred', and the third 'We are too frightened of making mistakes to use
the media to our advantage' (Ruddock 1991: 114–15).

MEETING THE MEDIA HEAD-ON

Martin Ruddock's conclusion, that social work (that is, local authority
social services) needs to be more pro-active in relations with the media,
had been regularly aired in the social work press since the late 1970s.
Articles have appeared by both media professionals and those delivering
social services; it is upon the latter category that I shall concentrate in the
main. At the centre of the genre is a debate about autonomy, although it
is rarely brought into sharp focus. Some writers assume that the press sets
the agenda, others that social work could if it were better organized or
seized the initiative.

One of the early reviews of media/social work relations, by Young,
followed on in *Social Work Today* (30 January 1979) from the 'Tragedies
revisited' series discussed earlier. Its analysis is complex and prescient,
showing an appropriate sense of *Realpolitik* from a 'former social work
committee chairman'. He opens with a strong assertion that, whatever
their imperfections, the news media are central to a democracy – although
it is important to grasp that all of them must make money, even if to cover
costs rather than generate profits. Young identifies the competitive
pressures that had – even by 1979 – increased the foregrounding of
'human interest' dimensions of issues. He also emphasizes the potential
of the local press with its 'greater inclination to print hand-outs from those
in authority'. Only his surprise that news media had not taken on the task
of educating the public about the 'claims and counter-claims of the
increasing number of professionals now occupying the expanded structure of government' seems to come from a more pastoral age.

During this period Geach was carrying out a study of 'the complete
national press cuttings on social work and social services from the
beginning of 1978 to August 1981' (*Community Care* 27 May 1982). He
makes the important point that, despite the subjective response of social
workers, 'they hardly get a press at all' even in the broadsheets. This, he
was told by a journalist, is because '"Social work is not a sexy subject. It
lacks glamour."' Geach adds to this the 'attitudes of many editors and
sub-editors', the profession's own inability to conceptualize its goals and
express them clearly, even in the context of an in-depth television series,
and a rigid interpretation of confidentiality. His solution is that social
work should invest 'more time and skill' in media relations, which does
not fit entirely convincingly with his blanket characterization of the

national press as preoccupied with the dramatic and sensational, prejudiced, and inappropriately staffed to deal with specialist issues.

Clode (*Social Work Today* 8 October 1984) also advocates social workers' taking the initiative, but targets local newspapers and broadcasts as the source of the '"good presses" which crop up sporadically'. Friendly relations with local media will, he suggests, yield two benefits: a willingness to publish department-generated 'good news' and the checking of unsolicited 'bad news' when it occurs. Unlike many commentators, Clode does not take the source of news stories as self-evident or arbitrary, but points out that members of the public with a grievance will seek to use media, with local outlets being much more accessible. This has since become even more salient as, for example, parents of children taken into care in Cleveland and elsewhere have set up self-help groups demonstrating considerable skills in news management (see Chapter 3 and Parton 1991: 197).

Guarded optimism is also the theme of Goldberg's review of press articles following the Jasmine Beckford furore (*Social Work Today* 25 April 1985). Sadly it is misplaced. No explanatory framework is offered for the positive coverage. The clichéd opening about the 'foaming, eye-gouging, snarling watchdog of public interests' and the assertion at the end, that populist-style columns in the mass tabloids (in this case Anne Robinson in the *Daily Mirror*) are mindless, suggests a pair of seriously flawed underlying assumptions: that news professionals are both autonomous and stupid. The author comments on a more-or-less supportive leader in the *Guardian* and follow-up letter, implying that these are unsurprising, but 'our old friend the *Daily Mail* . . . Even that newspaper went to some lengths to put the other side of the story.' But did it? The feature in question recounts the work of the NSPCC special unit in Manchester. This is not the state 'policing the family', but the voluntary sector and, lest the readers fear it could happen to them, we are talking about 'problem mothers and fathers'.

Reed's eye-catching article 'For social worker, read scapegoat' (*Community Care* 14 August 1986) also fails to move beyond an unreflective condemnation of journalistic practices. Having identified the fight for circulation and the tendency for important cases to be handled by crime reporters as key parameters, he goes on to ask why the 'standard scenario is then repeated'. His prescription is that the tendency for 'yet another one-sided story' will only end 'when the media show some interest in truly looking at social work or, more accurately, the society in which social workers work'. This would be limp from a social work practitioner, but for a NALGO national officer not to consider the effect of journalists' work routines and that newspapers operate in a capitalist market-place is either naïve or disingenuous.

Optimism is abundant in Dossett-Davies's call for the profession to 'stand up for itself' (*Community Care* 17 September 1987). A very experienced practitioner and 'member of the first BASW council', the author argues vehemently that the profession must learn to take pride in its achievements, both individually and collectively, and willingly accept that accountability sometimes means painful exposure. 'We have a great educational and propaganda war to win . . . we have not even *begun* to fight for our reputation and our profession' (his emphasis). The strategy is to be less secretive, clearer in communicating and – presumably – pro-active in dealing with the news media. Dossett-Davies does not address this in detail; his confidence about potential victory must come from an idealist (and idealistic) assumption that news agendas are set by rational argument and mutual understanding.

Social work's preoccupation with its media coverage seems to have peaked in 1987. In that year *Community Care* organized a training event, with supporting how-to booklet (Fry 1987). The advice is wide-ranging: 'Make sure you look the part', which, according to Fry (1987: 15), does not include senior management 'swigging beer from cans'. Conversely, at press conferences 'provide soft drinks too. (The drinking capacity of journalists is not always as great as assumed in social services circles)' (Fry 1987: 27). The different possibilities of local, national and specialist press and of broadcasting are considered, as is the distinction between news and features. Fry concludes: 'social services is now a very high-profile area and communicating with the media is, unavoidably, part of the senior manager's job' (1987: 49).

This call to seize the initiative was also the dominant theme of contemporary articles. Both Julia (*Community Care* 5 March 1987) and Grainger (*Community Care* 16 April 1987) describe their success in building relationships with the local press, in Kingston-upon-Thames and Slough respectively. Both stress the importance of meeting newspaper staff informally and having an organized, positive response to press approaches, even when the news is negative. The goal is to build a working relationship that will, on the one hand, sustain 'off-the-record' briefings which may contain or even eliminate adverse coverage and, on the other, ensure that 'good news' is well received. The extent of good relations is conveyed in Grainger's remark that 'When a social event, such as a staff retirement, took place, the local press would try to report it.' This is exactly the kind of undramatic, untitillating, comfortingly mundane, positive news that fills the local press. It mirrors some of the successful probation service news management described in Chapter 5.

Grainger and Julia imply that they have succeeded in influencing at least the local news agenda. Treacher (*Local Government Chronicle* 22 July 1988) reports his ordeal trying to keep some sort of control as Public Relations Officer for County Cleveland during the events of 1987–8. The extent of the coverage was staggering: '9,000 *press* cuttings accumulated in the first five weeks' in the PR department (my emphasis – broadcasting had apparently not been monitored). His 'lessons learned' were 'tight restrictions on who could talk to the press'; 'daily briefings for the key players'; providing model answers to likely questions; 'press conferences were tightly staged'; and television or radio interviews only agreed when the interviewer and any other participants were known. Treacher concludes that 'the story will continue to be aired for months, but after the past year's experiences the press office will cope with whatever the next twist will be'. Other accounts of the actual media coverage (for example Illsley 1989; Nava 1988) serve, however, as a reminder that, while sophisticated techniques of dealing with the news media are now necessary for social work agencies, they are not sufficient to ensure laudatory or even neutral treatment; the game is bigger and more complex than that.

SOCIAL WORKERS' UNDERSTANDING OF NEWS MEDIA AT WORK

Many of the articles described above are first-hand accounts, which gives them an appealing veracity. It does not guarantee their utility. The experiential needs to be interpreted from the conceptual, even though there is a long tradition in social work of resisting this.

First, many of the writers conflate extensive media exposure of an issue with public concern. Although free-market apologists for the more outrageous manifestations of the press will of course say that there is an axiomatic convergence between content and audience preferences, this is wholly contested. Even at the empirical level, Cohen (1973) and Hall *et al.* (1978) on moral panics and Schlesinger *et al.* (1991) on competition for resources in the criminal justice system demonstrate that the media and the control culture are frequently addressing each other for reasons of sectional interest and political advantage. 'The public' is marginal, its views only sought as they fit the pre-set discursive framework of *vox pop* television interviews and letters to the editor.

Ruddock invests the media/public relationship with an almost mystical – and certainly therapeutic – unity: 'I believe that society and the media needed me to make an honest acceptance of my responsibility before they were able to address the wider issues within the Kimberley Carlile debate' (Ruddock 1991: 115). Even when Hall *et al.* (1978) are most persuasive about the dominant ideology, they do not credit the media with this capacity for intentional action.

Most of the articles also adopt a mechanistic assumption of media effect, assuming that the audience will absorb their outputs uncritically. As we have seen in Chapter 1, one of the few points of agreement in contemporary media effect theory is that media messages are received through a complex filter of personal attributes, previous knowledge and social location.

A more prosaic, but nevertheless important, weakness in social work perspectives on the media (for example, 'Social Worker 2', Geach, Ruddock above) is a failure to distinguish between them, or having done so, to draw out the implications. Accounts of good coverage are almost all in relation to local media, but few consider why this should be so. Conversely, most of the distressed accounts of social work news relate to national media, but do not consider whether the more low-key, or even sympathetic approach, of local media (at least in the regions) may have an offsetting effect. Is the profession as London-centric as the national news media themselves?

Some commentators (for example Geach, Goldberg) treat the national press as monolithic, and yet the political alignment of newspapers is a key variable in determining their attitude to the welfare state and thus to the vicissitudes of local authority social services. Hostile coverage from the *Sun*, the *Daily Star* and the *Daily Mail* is recounted with horror, without taking account of the almost perfect coincidence of political and news values provided by a local authority scandal for a right-wing tabloid. For all its faults, the *Daily Mirror* bays for blood less often. The *Guardian* is expected to be understanding, but Goldberg (*Community Care* 25 April 1985) comments with surprise at a sympathetic feature in *The Times*. Here the different 'pitch' of a broadsheet newspaper modifies the effect of its political alignment.

Being a local authority social worker is inevitably to be 'at risk' of hostile treatment in Tory tabloid papers. Should practitioners not get some comfort from this and, through the contexualization, try to give it less significance as informed commentary on the quality of practice?

Some discussants of social work media treatment even elide all national media, press with broadcasting. Both the BBC and independent television and radio are statutorily barred from editorializing in news bulletins and must 'balance' the points of view expressed in documentary programmes. Detailed requirements for news and current affairs output are retained in the Broadcasting Act 1990. It is not pure chance that, for example, Ruddock felt better treated by broadcasters.

An extension of this tendency to deal with 'the media' as an undifferentiated bloc is failing to comprehend the commercial/fiscal, technical and organizational framework within which newsgathering occurs. Again, social workers appear trustingly to accept the 'as if' world of journalism, in which news is what the ace reporter has fought to uncover and the paper has published in the face of proprietorial and political pressure. As we have seen in Chapter 1, life is not like that for journalists, just as local authority social work is not giving grateful clients everything they need. Social workers, in short, show little awareness that news is manufactured from what is practicable and commercially safe. This includes the whole gamut from what is covered to what 'spin' is put on it according to the medium's style and market. Mass tabloids will, by definition, be concerned with the dramatic, quickly comprehended, personalized event, often within a strongly individualist political philosophy. The recourse to blaming individuals for things going wrong is hardly surprising.

Social workers writing about media coverage are frequently wanting media organizations not simply to be nicer, but to be what they cannot be. If the *Sun* started producing 2,500 word articles on the Social Chapter of the Maastricht Treaty it would not be the *Sun*. Nor can we expect the *Daily Mail* to become infused with a socialist feminist analysis of the family under capitalism.

Social workers sometimes fail to see journalists as employees in a complex system, doing a job more or less well. Ruddock seems surprised that television would want pictures of his entering the Kimberley Carlile public inquiry. It may have been insensitive to ask him to repeat it when they found no film in the camera, but it is hardly 'temerity' (Ruddock 1991: 111–12). This reaction stems from a failure by social work commentators on media behaviour to see themselves as part of a system too. Local authority social work is a public agency, so social workers are answerable to the public. This can be handled well or badly, with or without thoughtful management support, with or without vicious mass tabloid caricatures, but this accountability is not optional. The distinction between 'the public interest' and what is 'of interest to the public' is very controversial, and was fought out spectacularly during the summer of 1992 over the mass tabloids' treatment of the royal family's marital problems, and David Mellor's (then Secretary of State for the National Heritage) recreational arrangements. As a key witness in an official public inquiry, Martin Ruddock had stepped firmly into the domain of 'the public interest'.

Is it inappropriate for the local paper to headline an item 'MARIA WITNESS DIES IN HOSPITAL' (*Community Care* 9 January 1979)? Here was a senior figure in local government who had played an important part in a significant local event – and had died suddenly, in post, at a relatively young age. I suggest that this is of legitimate public interest and that to assume, as Shearer apparently does, that the local paper should have given priority to the 'grief of some of the people in headquarters' is unrealistic. So too is Papworth's claim that once he, too, had made himself public property by pressing criminal charges and appearing as chief witness in an Old Bailey trial (*Community Care* 16 July 1987) he should have had control over the inflection of news stories. It was tasteless and a distortion by the mass tabloids to treat a very frightening episode as a joke, but to deny them the right even to highlight its funnier aspects would, in other contexts, be described as censorship.

These dimensions of social work's perception of the news media are strikingly symmetrical with those aspects of news media professional ideology which contribute to its problem with social work. Both occupations seem to struggle to conceptualize their relationship in other than an individualist framework. For journalists this articulates with the myth of the macho, self-made, freebooting crusader discussed in Chapter 1. For social workers the ideal encounter with the news media would appear to be a quasi-therapeutic one-to-one meeting of minds, free of the baggage of diminishing resources, overbearing management, unpalatable policy strait-jackets, and even the obligations of electoral democracy. When criticizing their media treatment, social workers, as has been pointed out earlier, show a surprising lack of empathy and what the profession itself calls tendencies to 'omnipotence'. The mass tabloids want to know who did what, when, and why it went wrong, even if they do not start out searching for the 'bungler' surely behind every public sector mishap. They are little interested in policy or processes, but in events and persons. Even persons are dealt with as concretely as possible. What are their surface attributes? What have they done? Intentions and motivations are rarely of interest. When these come under scrutiny they, too, are simplified as Soothill and Walby (1991) describe of the construction of the 'sex fiend'. Why does this construction of issues as behaviour rather than processes and intentions cause social work particular problems?

THE AIMS AND VALUES OF SOCIAL WORK

In 1980 the then Secretary of State for Health and Social Services asked the National Institute for Social Work (NISW) to 'promote, at Government expense, an independent and authoritative enquiry into the role and tasks of social workers' (NISW 1982: vii). This was widely interpreted as a demand to justify the very existence of state social work by a radical right government disposed to reduce both the influence of local government and the size of the welfare state. Peter Barclay and his distinguished committee (of seventeen) succeeded: although the priorities and responsibilities of local authority social services were much altered during the 1980s, this was the result of wider policy change in areas like child protection, mental health, and the care of elderly people, not a frontal assault. The committee must have felt an enormous weight of responsibility for the future of a whole profession. Nevertheless, while they laid out what social workers were doing, they did not specify what the goals of the work might be. The main finding, that social workers' 'role and tasks' might be better streamlined under the twin heading of 'counselling' and 'social care planning', is actually a sophisticated analysis of means, not ends.

Even more significantly, given the stakes, the committee could not agree. Two minority reports were produced. One, signed by three members, wished to take the main report's endorsement of more community-based work further. The other dissentient, Robert Pinker, restated the core of social work as one-to-one social casework, with the apparent intention of having clearer and more achievable skills and goals for 'helping the client to manage his [sic] own life' (NISW 1982: 239).

The British Association of Social Workers (BASW) has only about one-third of local authority staff in membership, but in the absence of any real competitor it tries to speak for social workers outside the probation service (for whom NAPO is both trade union and professional association). In 1977 BASW published a code of ethics, which was revisited and evaluated in a book of essays published in 1985 (Watson 1985). One of the authors opens his chapter with the assertion 'It is very understandable that the code avoided defining social work' (Leighton 1985: 60) and goes on to endorse a pragmatic approach: social work is what social workers do.

This is an interpretation shared by Bamford although not with approval. His analysis of *The Future of Social Work* (1990) starts with a comprehensive catalogue of what went wrong in the recent past: the reorganization following the Seebohm report (Cmnd 3703 1968) should have been the launch pad for the consolidation of the profession. Instead, the failure of social work to achieve its professional aspirations of self-regulation in terms of training and disciplinary action against professional failings encapsulated the failure of social work as a whole to reach agreement on its role and function.

(Bamford 1990: xi)

This faith in the benefits of licensing is disputed among social workers. What is more salient is that a senior practitioner, who has been chair of BASW, could assert in 1990 that the goals of social work were not agreed.

Further evidence of the difficulty in specifying goals and therefore – crucially – what might constitute 'success' comes from the 'Rules and Requirements for the Diploma in Social Work' (CCETSW 1991). This is the formal statement of the new framework for approving qualifying courses for social workers, whether in social services, the probation service or the voluntary or private sector. Arriving at this point had taken over a decade of Byzantine manoeuvring. (See Bamford (1990) for the story until the late 1980s.) CCETSW is a government-funded quango and has been struggling for more cash to be allocated to lengthen the Diploma in Social Work (DipSW) and to provide training for the legions of other staff who work in domiciliary and residential care. Both aims are widely agreed to be vital. Again there is heavy political pressure to be assertive and compelling: the stakes are high. The opening definition reads:

Social work is an accountable professional activity with enables individuals, families and groups to identify personal, social and environmental difficulties adversely affecting them. Social work enables them to manage these difficulties through supportive, rehabilitative, protective or corrective action. Social work promotes social welfare and responds to wider social needs promoting equal opportunities ... Social work has the responsibility to protect the vulnerable and exercise authority under statute.

(CCETSW 1991: 8)

Even accepting the importance attached to 'empowerment' in contemporary social work thinking, it is hard not to reflect that these are still means or, at best, middle-order goals rather than end goals.

Intertwined with the lack of consensus about goals is wide variation in the means themselves. It is not merely that there is an attractive menu of methods on offer, but that workers seem unsure of the techniques' potential and how to conceptualize people's 'personal, social and environmental difficulties' so as to guide their choice. Parsloe and Stevenson (DHSS 1978) undertook a detailed review of social services field workers' understanding and use of a range of discrete intervention techniques. They conclude:

> On the whole, our respondents' descriptions of their work did not suggest that practice was drawn from specific theoretical perspectives. It may be that they had so internalised theory that they put it into practice without being conscious of it or being able to talk about it . . . There was some evidence that many of the experienced workers were accustomed to working mainly at an intuitive level . . . Most social workers were diffident about claiming success in their work with clients. In many cases they acknowledged that results came very slowly – if at all.
>
> (DHSS 1978: 134–6)

The situation seems little changed since this work was done in the mid-1970s – not that the spending cuts, political pressures and the avalanche of statutes in the 1980s made professional reflection and regrouping very likely. Coulshed's introductory text (1991) discusses a range of methods (task-centred, psychosocial, family work, etc.). She acknowledges difficulties caused by competing paradigms of the social world and therefore of appropriate techniques for change, points out the risks of slavish adherence to one method and of atheoretical practicality – and stoutly rebuts the idea that theorization reduces spontaneity. Again, it is less the message than the medium which is interesting. This is the second edition of a book in a BASW series, suggesting a text that is both authoritative and useful. Nevertheless, Coulshed is not offering students clear directions, but the tools for thoughtful eclecticism. This may well be both realistic and intellectually healthy given the problems which social workers must face – but is it reassuring?

In reality, if social workers were to deconstruct their 'intuition' they would find a large part based on the skills of forming and using one-to-one relationships. Parsloe and Stevenson (DHSS 1978) discovered that, by default, most of their respondents were using intervention techniques loosely called 'casework'. Avenues to change based on group functioning or community-based collective action were rare. Even specific models of work with individuals, like task-centred work or the identification of an explicit 'contract', were poorly understood. Ways of working were attributed to common sense. But the casework was not 'narrowly directed to discussing the client's emotional functioning or interpersonal relationships' (DHSS 1978: 133) derived from a psychopathological model of the self. Rather, the relationship skills were often deployed in indirect work on behalf of clients, with fuel boards, housing authorities or colleagues, for example.

The same skill is given prominence in the Barclay report (NISW 1982), where counselling is described as:

> the activity which social workers themselves have traditionally regarded as the hallmark of their calling; and which several of our respondents consider to lie at the core of social work . . . we believe it is essential that social workers continue to be able to provide counselling and we use the word to cover a range of activities in which an attempt is made to understand the meaning of some event or state of being to an individual, family or group.
>
> (NISW 1982: 41)

Robert Pinker goes further. For him 'social casework' is the 'fundamentally distinctive method of social work . . . In my view, therefore, social work and social casework are virtually synonymous, but my definition of social casework is a broad one which includes counselling and various practical tasks' (NISW 1982: 239).

In different ways, Parsloe and Stevenson, the Barclay committee majority, and Pinker are all preoccupied with finding a realistic accommodation between social work's service to clients, workers' relationship to their local authority employers, and that between local authority and central government. They are willing to be reasonably pragmatic about the framing of much social work endeavour by the state: the point is to do it with efficiency and clarity of purpose, but without loss of humanity and concern for clients. Hence the quasi-scientific search for better tools and more easily defined outcomes.

All this is anathema to Hugh England (1986) who wants to reinstate social work as creative, an 'art'. Social workers may not be able to 'prove' in a positivist sense that they are helping but 'Good social workers *know* (England 1986: 4; his emphasis). England wants social work to be skilful, effective and purposeful but defined by the relationship between worker and client, not driven by the latest government circular – or research in social policy or psychology. For him, 'intuition' is not to be derided as a mush of unidentified ideology, but refined. Needless to add, the one-to-one casework or counselling relationship is even more pivotal in his approach than in the official/political defences of social work discussed above.

In the 1970s there was an active radical social work movement (see for example Bolger *et al.* 1981; Corrigan and Leonard 1978). This not only located the true aetiology of personal problems in the socio-political structure but advocated community-based collective action as the logical intervention style. The fiscal and morale problems of state social work in the 1980s have made the radical critique hard to implement. In effect, innovation in practice has been scaled down to the exploration of family- and group-based techniques.

SOCIAL WORK AS 'EMOTIONAL LABOUR'

If there was ever any doubt that social work is 'emotional labour', the restoration of relationship work to the centre of practice has dispelled it. James (1989) defines emotional labour as the 'social regulation of feeling' – much of it done by women in the family, unpaid. This does not, of course, mean that it does not produce value. Emotional work in the home is an essential part of the family as reproducer of labour power. But emotional labour also occurs in the public domain 'undefined, unexplained, usually unrecorded', again predominantly undertaken by women, underpaid. The burden of this demanding work is often carried by the lowest-ranking staff. In James's discussion of a hospice she observes that medical staff will tell the patient that they are dying, leaving front-line staff like nursing auxiliaries to try and cope with the emotional response. Their time is assumed to be more flexible, their skills not 'skills' but 'natural' in a woman. Presumably the same could be observed in any residential care home.

In schools, too, the emotional dimension of the work is expanding as teachers take on more pastoral care. Again, as Walters (1991) points out, there is ambivalence about whether this is 'real' work. Like 'special needs', there is a tendency for the delivery and management of pastoral care to be done by women staff while men take posts related to academic knowledge and administration. (And not just in schools.)

James, Walters and other recent British studies of emotional labour have scrutinized public sector employment. The classic initial study (Russell Hochschild 1983), however, was based on a US private-sector employer and develops rather different emphases. The core of Russell Hochschild's book is about the training of Delta Airlines' cabin staff to produce the kind of soothing, quasi-domestic atmosphere that is essential for a successful commercial airline. Not only do passengers' anxieties have to be subdued (even when talking about safety procedures), but the level of in-flight comfort is one of the few differentiating factors in a very uniform commodity. Candidates were initially selected on the basis of personal qualities: 'a certain kind of outgoing middle-class sociability'

(Russell Hochschild 1983: 97) – which is remarkably like the qualities of the 'angels' recruited to nursing by the 'good' London teaching hospital described by Smith (1992). The key difference is that learning to manage emotions is the centre of the Delta Airlines' training but picked up along the way in the hospital. 'The lessons were in deep acting – acting "as if the cabin is your home" and "as if this passenger has a traumatic past"' – the latter being the way to handle 'irates' (Russell Hochschild 1983: 120). She reports that even when staff knew they had learned these techniques, knew why, and discussed their effectiveness, they could feel guilty about acting, thus showing a breakdown of '"healthy" estrangement' from the job (Russell Hochschild 1983: 188). The company had bought part of the private self to extract profit.

James (1989) and Smith (1992) on health care and Walters (1991) on teaching all underline, in contrast, that staff doing emotional work are rarely given any systematic training, even though the personal cost is known. New thinking about the 'nursing process', putting the nurse/patient relationship centre-stage as part of a 'holistic' approach, still relies upon the student nurse's constructing these interpersonal skills from her/his own experience and the example of senior staff who grasp the implications of the shift in style (Smith 1992).

When the burden becomes too much, nursing and teaching have refuges in common: technology and routine. Real knowledge in nursing is still stubbornly conceptualized as technical/medical. Thus an experienced and dedicated psychiatric nurse could still wistfully regard acute surgical nursing to be 'real work' (Smith 1992: 57). Even where the rigidities of old-style hospital wards have been softened, there is still an endless round of practical things to do. More diffuse care for patients can be expressed through non-essentials like hair-washing and nail-cutting. In teaching too there is a reassuring impersonal structure of timetable and lessons. While distance from the role may not be a very comfortable long-term strategy, boredom, irritation and weariness can be concealed by a well-prepared lesson and a polished 'turn'. Teachers may even hone a slightly alienated and caricatured professional persona in order to keep order and get their subject across.

Social workers do not have the same possibilities of 'going through the motions' while they recoup their emotional energy. In part this is because of the diversity of situations they face, in part because of the lack of consensus about both means and ends discussed above. More than that, their vulnerability to the demands of emotional work derives from the ideology of the casework relationship which, as we have seen above, remains at the centre of the job.

Take, for example, Keith Lucas's standard text *Giving and Taking Help* (1972). This is clearly intended to be non-sectarian and not professionally precious. 'Anyone ought to be able to help' (Keith Lucas 1972: 71) with the right motivation and training in the essential skills of 'reality', 'support' and 'empathy'.

> I have spoken of 'empathy' as an emotion and rightly so . . . It always involves the ability to enter into this feeling, to experience it and therefore to know its meaning for another person . . . an assurance of feeling can only be communicated if the feeling actually exists.
>
> (Keith Lucas 1972: 81–2)

Despite his early assertion that most people have the capacity to be successful 'helpers', Keith Lucas has a chapter on the personal qualities which will predispose to success.

Keith Lucas cannot be written off as a classic from a bygone age, as those people who now occupy senior practice and management posts in social work were trained when it was in current use. What of texts which will have influenced more recent entrants to the profession? Martin Davies's *The Essential Social Worker* (1981) might well have been titled 'the no-nonsense social worker'. He is bitterly critical of what he sees as the hubris of social work in the 1960s and 1970s, and of the political posturing of radical social work. For Davies social work should be more practical in every way. It should codify its methods and teach them more concretely; it should be realistic about the constraints of state bureaucracy; it should accept that many other occupations inhabit the same territory, and it should accept that any 'change' achieved will be modest in most situations: 'The social worker couldn't make it worse because it couldn't *be* worse' (Davies 1981: 116; his emphasis). But the brisk practicality does not eliminate the focus on the self. 'Social work is the structure *and* the person' (Davies 1981: 156; his emphasis), he asserts, and moves on to listing positive and negative personal attributes for social work practice, citing, *inter alia*, Keith Lucas. He concludes with his own compilation:

> First, it must be said again, come Truax and Carkhuff's recommended qualities for counsellors: genuineness, empathy and warmth – plus persuasiveness . . . [which] do appear to be essential to *good* social work . . . Each social worker is a unique being and it follows from this that the use of self is one crucial part of his function [and] that the development of self is a significant strategy in its own right.
>
> (Davies 1981: 159–60)

Naturally, given his general orientation, England locates 'use of self' at the heart of social work:

> the task which is required of the helper . . .is as if the helper must make a journey with the client ... The worker has to 'live' his understanding; to fail to do so is not only hypocrisy and bad faith, but the frustration of his healing ambitions.
>
> (England 1986: 23, 31)

Part One of *Social Work as Art* (five chapters) is called 'The Problem of the Use of Self' (England 1986). By this England means how to identify, retrieve and cultivate those aspects of the self which are necessary for good practice. He does not write about the use of self as having a cost for the worker.

A survey of practitioner attitudes by Holme and Maizels (1978: 58) confirmed this orientation. 'In commenting on the factors which they felt were the most helpful to their effectiveness [workers] ... tended to emphasize above all some aspect of their personal qualities.'

How does this help to understand the sensitivity of social work to its news media coverage? To draw together the points made so far: first, there is apparently widespread agreement that social work is about 'the use of the self'. The cost of being an 'emotional labourer' is constantly acknowledged but dealt with through the relatively informal medium of supervision in training and at work, and by colleague support. While these may be consoling, it is at least questionable whether they do not further – and counter-productively – reinforce the deeply held professional value about authenticity. England (1986: 31) is clear that the emotional response to the client must somehow be real. Diana Lees (*Community Care* 9 January 1991) wrote 'it was an effort to care', not 'it was an effort to be able to behave as if I cared'. Even Davies, the bracing pragmatist, hesitates. He argues that being friendly is not the same as being a friend and that 'warmth of manner' (1981: 20) is part of the professional persona which is both necessary and well understood by clients. 'There is clearly *an element of acting in this*, but the performance emerges as crucial to good social work in the eyes of the client. Professionalism is the projection of a concerned interest in the client's welfare' (Davies 1981: 20; my emphasis).

So acting is out. Nursing, teaching and even Delta Airlines have two further advantages, as we have seen: first, the safety net of routine for the tired, harassed or disillusioned worker. Second, there is some achievable concept of 'success'. For an airline the criteria are relatively straight-forward; in health care the social definition of health has been captured by powerful players (see Chapter 8 on the idea of a profession); in schools 'success' is now highly politicized, but the battle is over different definitions, not the search for it.

In social work, by contrast, the concentration on use of self and the pivotal nature of the relationship with the client means that social workers are offering themselves unmediated and unprotected as both tool and goal. An almost complete homology has been constructed between the job and the person. Clergy find themselves in the same exposed position. The implication of this dilemma for the Christian church emerged in the fourth century when the Donatist schism developed, based on the belief that the validity of sacraments is mediated by the holiness or otherwise of the person administering them (*Oxford Dictionary of the Christian Church*). This heresy is briskly disposed of in Article Twenty-Six of the Church of England: 'Of the Unworthiness of the Minister which hinders not the effect of the Sacrament' (*Book of Common Prayer* 1662). The problem for social workers is that, given the problems of defining their goals and demonstrating that they have been achieved, it is almost impossible to detach themselves from the 'sacrament' that they are offering. How does this explain the reaction of social workers – particularly those in social services – to adverse media coverage? I would argue that the identification of the self with the job means that criticism is experienced as a deeply personal rejection, especially if colleague and employer support seems to have failed too, as for Martin Ruddock after the Kimberley Carlile case.

It also has collective consequences. Fry, writing as a journalist specializing in social work, comments that the profession's 'obsessive craving for the laudatory is unrealistic' (1991: 66). Satyamurti (1981), a psychiatric social worker become researcher on 'occupational survival', describes the amount of energy poured into creating and maintaining team- or office-based solidarity, amounting to a siege mentality. This is in part sustained by the projection of negative characteristics on those who threaten the world view created: administrators, management, other professionals – even clients. Surely this applies *a fortiori* to the news media?

Closing ranks is a familiar part of handling difficult work. As Hughes classically observed in 'Mistakes at work': 'those who are subject to the same risks will compose a collective rationale which they whistle to one another to keep up their courage and they will build up collective defenses against the lay world' (Hughes 1971: 318). This can provide comfort but it will not necessarily benefit the profession, clients or others in the arena in which it operates. It has even proved difficult for social work to establish solidarity at other than the face-to-face level of team or office. The fragmentary nature of the profession and the effect of the lack of unity on its knowledge base and capacity for joint action are among the issues considered in the following chapter.

Chapter 8

Professions, the state and social work

The edginess about social work's media coverage is both personal and political. On the one hand practitioners and managers fear that the next furore will spotlight their department, their own team. It could even be their own face in the photograph beneath the accusing headline. At the same time, adverse media coverage is taken as an index of the poor public standing of the profession as a whole. Attempts at explanation by social work insiders have, as we have seen, blamed media values and practices, or have accused the social work profession itself of poor self-presentation. This inability to present a better image is in turn explained by the alleged characteristics of social workers themselves, how the profession is organized, who dictates its aims and methods, and the lack of accurate public knowledge of, in the Barclay Committee's phrase, social work's 'rôle and tasks' (NISW 1982).

In this chapter I shall examine four dimensions of social work in society: its relation to the welfare state since 1979; what it means for an occupation to be 'a profession' and the implications of this for social work; how association with the feminine and feminized world of 'caring' affects social work in the public arena; and what might be the interaction between media treatment and lack of direct public experience of social work.

GOVERNMENT AND WELFARE IN THE 1980s

Pressure on welfare expenditure did not arrive suddenly with Margaret Thatcher's government in 1979. During the 1970s both Conservative and Labour governments had struggled with the mounting fiscal problems of the UK, where long-term economic decline was intensified by the world-wide financial lurch caused by the oil crisis of 1973. Inflation became the shared preoccupation of politicians and public. The solution offered by both Tory and Labour governments was to cut public expenditure. Labour's most savage critics came from the radical left: the Counter Information Services/Community Development Project's *Cutting the Welfare State* (CIS/CDP 1975) is a quintessential example. Hall *et al.* (1978 (see Chapter 1)) characterize the whole period as a 'legitimation crisis' in which the state's ability to ensure the consent of the population through the expectation of modest relative affluence faltered. Instead, actually or potentially disruptive groups like the unemployed and political or trade union activists had to be contained by legal sanctions. The Glasgow University Media Group's first study (1976) is an account of the domination of television news in the mid-1970s by inflation, service cuts and the consequent industrial unrest. Another specific outcome was the spotlight on the cost of benefits, not only in the UK but in other developed societies. This particularly targeted those payments to able-bodied adults, like unemployment and (then) supplementary benefit, and was symbolized in the media 'scrounger-phobia' charted by Golding and Middleton (1982).

The shock of the 1970s cuts in welfare provision was precisely that they were unforeseen, piecemeal, and indicated the collapse of a set of broad policy assumptions shared by both the one-nation Tory and the centre-left Labour governments of the post-war period. Here were governments going against a whole edifice of implicit and explicit social commitments. Not so the 1979 Conservative government under Mrs Thatcher: the platform was a radical right version of freedom where the individual and his/her family are free to make their own way within the enabling framework of a strong state regulated by the market and the law. After more than a decade's hindsight the cruel inadequacies of this philosophy and the gulf between the rhetoric and the reality are beginning to be coolly analysed. (In respect of social policy and welfare, see the useful overviews by Johnson (1990) and Manning and Page (1992).)

One could argue that a characteristic of the entire post-1979 era has been a clouding of the very idea of a distinction between rhetoric and reality. We have entered post-modern politics and policy-making. Presentation is much more important than content. Policies are implemented with little consideration of practicality (the community charge/poll tax being the most high-profile débâcle). Public expenditure priorities are determined not by analysis or local accountability, but in the quasi-market-place of a media shouting match; see Schlesinger *et al.* (1991) on this contest over criminal justice issues – all of which makes the news media an even more engrossing subject of study.

Much of this rhetoric was generated by a succession of right-wing 'think-tanks'. Even if, in the post-Thatcher revisionism, some of their prominent members started to question how much had really changed, their output alarmed those in their sights. Not only was the content threatening, but the Thatcher government's imperviousness to argument made effective ripostes hard to mount. One of the most consistently influential radical right lobbies has been in respect of education; social work and welfare have not had the same organized critique. (Why not would be a fascinating topic for policy analysis in itself, given the potential of the target.)

The nearest to the education 'Black Papers' was the publication in 1980 of Brewer and Lait's *Can Social Work Survive?* At the time its arguments about local authority social services departments were seen as potentially representing the philosophy of the new government. Even Brewer and Lait's format embodies 'Victorian values': the chapters have italicized epigraphs summarizing what follows; the language is ponderous, the style simultaneously arch and reminiscent of a nineteenth-century pamphleteer. The book's argument rests on two assumptions. First, that social work practice is largely 'casework', not in the eclectic sense demonstrated by Parsloe and Stevenson and the Barclay Committee and discussed above, but that social workers actually attempt individual psychotherapy. Second, despite recurrent calls for better research into the effectiveness of social work, Brewer and Lait are quite content to assert, on the basis of hearsay evidence, that the social work strikes of the late 1970s showed the lack of effect of social work. The authors call, in the mode of disinterested pursuit of evidence, for a 'royal commission or committee of enquiry' (Brewer and Lait 1980: 196) to be set up, but their preferred solution is settled. Social work should become a subordinate occupation within health care. Failing that, they argue that it could be reduced to a set of purely practical bureaucratic tasks within local government, for which only 'apprenticeship' would be required. Those practitioners and trainers who felt that social work and its methods added up to more should go into private practice: 'It may be that casework-trained social workers have skills marketable to middle-class neurotics' (Brewer and Lait 1980: 203). Although the publication of the book post-dated the setting up of the Barclay Committee, one must assume that the case within it had been pressed upon Conservative politicians; they had already been trailed by Lait in two 1979 *Community Care* articles.

Yet social work has survived and the book is almost forgotten. How could this happen to a service so bound up with the 'dependency culture' that was also one of the biggest spending departments in the hated local government, the epitome of what Mrs Thatcher called 'drooling and drivelling' about caring? The answer, apart from the reality gap referred to above is that, during the 1980s, local authority social work – and probation – have been changed. As in other areas of the public sector like higher education, practitioners find themselves offering a service which is apparently the same but has an altered statutory basis and moral justification. This has partly been achieved by the application of the 'disciplines' imposed elsewhere: the promotion of internal markets; managerialist techniques of reduced job security, sidelining of collective agreements, performance-related pay, devolved budgets, and mechanisms in search of 'quality' once it has become questionable; direct cuts in expenditure; and – crucially for social services – the systematic weakening of local government through restrictions on revenue-raising and other powers. Everywhere, whatever the philosophy of the party in power locally, services have been reduced or hived off, jobs lost and morale shattered. As Wilding (1992) points out in his summing up of the decade, the very ideas of collective provision and of the public sector as mitigating social inequality have been profoundly undermined.

During the 1980s, two processes transformed local authority social services and the probation service: the concentration of effort in a limited number of areas and the ring-fencing of practice by statute. For the probation service the choice was stark: abandon most of the stuff about client needs and rehabilitation, start talking (at least in public) about retribution, recompense and punishment, or be marginalized by a new agency aimed at delivering 'punishment in the community'. These changes are discussed in more detail in Chapter 5.

All three main areas of social services' responsibility – child care, the provision of services for elderly people, and work with mentally ill people – have been reconstructed. In 1983 the Mental Health Act confirmed social workers' role in the care of mentally ill people, but required that the duties be carried out by specialist workers who had acquired in-service qualification as an 'approved social worker'.

Longer life expectation combined with a falling birthrate has greatly increased the projected proportion of elderly people in the UK population. This is not by itself a 'problem' but has become a major political and policy issue because of the potential cost of providing residential care for the growing number who are very old and frail, within a context of attempts to limit public expenditure. (See Phillipson (1992) for a fuller discussion.) The solution, for elderly people and people with a mental illness or learning difficulty, was seen to lie in 'community care' and a committee under Sir Roy Griffiths set up to advise the Secretary of State. As Norman Johnson explains, Griffiths envisaged local authorities in the key 'enabling' functions of assessing overall community needs; financial management of community care funds; monitoring of performance; provision of information; and assessment of individual needs (Johnson 1990: 164, summarizing Griffiths 1988). 'Under these arrangements, social workers would become case managers, designing packages aimed at achieving the most effective combination of services within the resources available' (Johnson 1990: 164).

The whole concept depended upon a large transfer to local authorities of funds for residential provision previously directly under the control of the Department of Social Security. This was not congenial to Mrs Thatcher. Nevertheless it went into the White Paper (Cm 849 1989) and subsequent legislation. 'When the provisions of the NHS and Community Care Act 1990 are fully implemented . . . local authority social service departments will be changed out of all recognition' (Johnson 1990: 183). Growing alarm was being expressed at the size of the likely shortfall between assessed needs and cash available even before the Act came into force in April 1993 – a date which was already a postponement. Social services staff face a changed task and new skills are required. There are some central funds available for in-service training, but little sign that these new demands have been incorporated into the guidelines for the new DipSW (CCETSW 1991).

The lack of public debate on community care contrasts sharply with two decades of controversy about child protection, which overshadows all other aspects of social work training, practice and organization. As in 'care in the community', social services departments find themselves still in the lead role, but with the greater responsibility has come decreased autonomy. Parton (1991), in his authoritative study, maps the reconstruction of 'child abuse' into 'child protection' in the 1980s. (See also Parton (1985) for the earlier stages of the process.) Two potentially contradictory forces have been in play. First, the renewed political emphasis on the privacy of family life in which parents have duties to support and control children (and support their own parents) but a reciprocal right to resist outside interference. This has been central to the radical right philosophy of an individualist, consumption-led society, where even citizenship becomes commodified as consumerism. If, however, the family is to fulfil its task of reproducing the labour force, and even reincorporate some of the work of caring for those who are dependent because of young or old age, sickness or disability, there must be a frontier of acceptable behaviour, beyond which legal sanctions can be invoked. This would suggest the kind of 'army of snoopers' paraded by right-wing tabloids to deride the public sector. The philosophers' stone is to isolate the 'really' deviant: the scroungers among claimants; the violent offender; the dangerously mentally ill – and the potentially abusive parent.

All these categories are, of course, axiomatically a manageable minority. 'In theory the identification of the dangerous individual or family would provide the mechanism for both ensuring that children are protected while also avoiding unwarrantable interventions' (Parton 1991: 198). Thus the technology of detecting and preventing child abuse becomes more and more ambitious, detailed and prescriptive (Dingwall 1989), surrounded by ramparts of DoH and local guidelines and manuals. Simultaneously, areas of social work discretion over parental rights have been transferred, in the 1989 Children Act, to the civil courts. The Act also confers on parents greater legal rights to challenge social work decisions (see Parton 1991, and Stevenson 1989 for full details).

Parton's account of the growth of the professional discourse on 'dangerousness' and the recasting of professional decision-making during the 1980s links together developments not only in child protection, but in mental health and criminal justice too. Social work survives, but under a new regime of legalism which is:

> evidence of the collapse of the political consensus upon which the institutional fabric of the welfare state was so dependent and the development of an influential liberal individualist critique of the professionalised paternalism and bureaucratic decision-making which seemed to characterise local authority social work.
>
> (Parton 1991: 195)

SOCIAL WORK AND PROFESSIONAL POWER

Social workers are still profoundly split over the pursuit of 'professionalism'. Those in favour justify it as benefiting clients through improved standards of practice and more clout with other key occupational groups. Those against condemn the whole concept as élitist, exclusionary and a direct contradiction of the concern with fighting inequality so central to social work that it is embodied in the training rules (CCETSW 1991). Academic debate is similarly divided about the moral claims of 'professions'. From the mid-1970s the notion of 'professionalism' as a discrete social formation was rejected and the concept folded into the wider debate on social stratification and occupational control. (See, for example, Johnson 1972, 1977; Parkin 1979; a very useful summary by Witz 1992.) Claims to client-orientated service were dismissed and professions reclassified simply as a particularly effective way of defending occupational interests. This is the position taken by Sarfatti Larson who states bluntly:

> Professionalism is thus an attempt to translate one order of scarce resources – special knowledge and skills – into another – social and economic rewards . . . Anti-market and anti-capitalist principles were incorporated in the professions' task of organizing for a market because they were elements which supported social credit and the public's belief in professional ethicality.
>
> (Sarfatti Larson 1977: vii, 63)

The profession, in short, is pursuing the benefits of monopoly control.

Recently there have been signs of reconsideration. Halliday, for example, rejects this 'implicit narcissism' (1987: 3), with its focus entirely on economic reward, the pursuit of group upward social mobility, and the consolidation of class position. He takes much more seriously the professional claim to an expert esoteric knowledge that can only be evaluated by peers and thus requires a code of professional ethics in place of *caveat emptor*: 'licensure may have protected the gullible from exploitation and personal tragedy' (Halliday 1987: 350). Professional institutions may incidentally confer market advantage, but this is better understood as an outcome of the 'professional project', rather than a deliberate collective strategy. Once an occupation has acquired legal protections it can, as it were, relax since it is 'less occupationally vulnerable, less reflexively self-protective and pre-occupied' (Halliday 1987: 353). At that point it can step down its lobbying and public relations activities and, he implies, focus on the 'real work'. Halliday's general position, then, is to situate professions as one – albeit very effective – type of interest group in a plural society. In his study, which centres on US lawyers, professional privilege is a tacit contract with government, which, in a highly differentiated society, has to delegate key functions. Professional organization is one way of meeting the potential crisis of 'ungovernability' (Halliday 1987: 4).

Alongside these opposing interpretations of the significance of the search for professional status are, though, important areas of agreement. The first is that there is no standard list of attributes which, once acquired, turns an occupation into a profession. Johnson (1972) very effectively dismantled this 'trait model', arguing that the professional project is neither unilinear nor ahistorical, like the climbing of a widely recognized ladder, where only the top rung is 'success'. It is the acquisition, to a greater or lesser extent, and through varying combinations of circumstances, of the capacity to control a range of key aspects of work: the choice of techniques and their development; the selection and training process; the licensing (and unlicensing) of practitioners; the determination of the nature of the service to be offered and to whom.

Second, there is not now seen to be any fundamental opposition between being 'professional' and working in a bureaucratic organization (Sarfatti Larson 1977; Freidson 1986). What is interesting is how the competing demands are managed, which in turn relates to the profession's power in the market derived from the demand for its expertise. In how many professions today are the majority of practitioners in small, genuinely self-employed groups? One of the few in the UK is veterinary medicine, of which one might ask, with Freidson (1986: 122), where is the joy in self-employment? Freidson uses US school teachers as his example of professionals in a bureaucracy. While accepting the over-arching control of the state, both centrally and locally, he sees teachers as 'In essence brokers between policies established from above and the concrete conduct of the classroom' (Freidson 1986: 162). This is reminiscent of Terence Johnson's (1972) argument that 'state mediated' professions like social work have considerable operating space as a result of their guaranteed flow of clients and the privacy of the professional encounter: a key point to which we shall return.

The third and crucial area of agreement between theorists on the professions is that a core body of distinctive knowledge is essential to the professional project. 'Cognitive commonality, however minimal, is indispensable if professionals are to coalesce into an effective group' says Sarfatti Larson (1977: 40), who goes on to describe a chain from codification through 'depersonalization' of knowledge to the culminating claim to be 'objective'. 'A scientific basis stamps the professional himself with the legitimacy of the general body of knowledge and a mode of cognition, the epistemological superiority of which is taken for granted in our society' (Sarfatti Larson 1977: 41). While Sarfatti Larson assumes that this knowledge is merely a means to the end of monopoly power, and writers like Halliday are more accepting of claims to expertise, there is no disagreement that a profession must 'establish its expert credentials' (Halliday 1987: 45). Ironically, once achieved, one of the hallmarks of the successful professional group is that it can increase the ratio of 'indeterminacy' to 'technicality' (Jamous and Peloille 1970). Where the occupation controls entry, training and licensing, mystification of the 'art' of medical diagnosis, or of the capacity of the architect to 'create' rather than specify a list of components, or of the unique alchemy of the client/practitioner relationship, is an important exclusionary mechanism.

Pace England (1986), justifications based on intuition and the special personal qualities of practitioners – 'virtualities' (Jamous and Peloille 1970) – can only be used when a group has a power-base; they are not the foundation upon which to build one. Central to this is control not only of licensing, subject of so much social work aspiration, but also of the training process. Sarfatti Larson, Freidson and Halliday all emphasize the importance of 'the modern university' in refining, elaborating and reproducing professional expertise, once established. Here a vital accommodation between the occupation and society takes place. The institutional structures of universities confer legitimacy on the type and level of knowledge acquired by invoking ideas of academic freedom and the disinterested pursuit of learning yet in powerful professions the validation of qualifying courses will be heavily influenced or even completely controlled by professional associations. Since eminent researchers and academics will probably sit alongside distinguished practitioners in the professional association, the circle will be complete.

This tidy scenario does not, as we have seen in the previous chapter, characterize contemporary UK social work. Attempts to define goals by both BASW and CCETSW have had to be pitched at such levels of generality that any unifying potential disappears. In order to validate training courses CCETSW has had to prescribe the necessary values, knowledge and skills for practice. Even after the attempt to bridge the goals/methods gap by specifying 'competencies', the essence of social work remains elusive. Many of the competencies deal with scene-setting for intervention: assessment, planning, evaluation, being a responsible professional. Criticism of the lack of preparedness of newly qualified workers has produced the concept of 'areas of particular practice', and yet the rules do not specify them, still less which permutation of knowledge and intervention techniques might be relevant. The nearest approximation to consensus in social work is that one-to-one relationship skills are vital (although these too come in competing paradigms). Even this is not privileged in the framework for training.

It could be argued that this cognitive anarchy is a realistic reflection of social work's location at the nub of the most contested parts of social life, especially given its reliance on knowledge from the social sciences, which do not – or cannot, depending upon your theoretical persuasion – provide a strong technological basis. Yet there are many examples of well-established occupations which do not rely upon a positivist justification of their knowledge base: Halliday (1987) uses the military as an example; the nascent professionalization of policing is another.

The problem, I would argue, is not inherent in the social work task. By a paradox, this continued fragmentation of the cognitive base comes, rather, from an artificially monolithic occupational structure. The Seebohm-inspired reforms of the early 1970s (Cmnd 3703 1968) brought together workers from the old child care, mental health and welfare local authority departments with psychiatric social workers and hospital almoners, leaving only the probation service and workers for the voluntary sector outside. (See Parry and Parry 1979, for a full account.) It has been a matter of dispute for the last twenty years whether Seebohm's intention was that the proposed one-stop family service would be provided by multi-skilled teams or whether all workers would be multi- skilled. At all events, the setting up of a common pattern of training further entrenched the concept of generic skills, which is how we arrived at the encompassing but unspecific list proposed in the DipSW 'Rules and Requirements' (CCETSW 1991). Even pre-Seebohm, many in the profession apparently expected that common training would consolidate generic skills, thus speeding the formation of a single cohesive professional grouping, able to pursue a more successful project (Parry and Parry 1979).

But achieving consensus about technique assumes an agreed definition of the task. Both before and since Seebohm the state has been the major consumer of social work and has largely determined its activities. Arguably, however, when those activities took place in single-purpose agencies, there was some potential for developing common understanding about relevant knowledge and skills. The setting up of post-Seebohm departments has, effectively, meant that 'social work' has become a large portfolio of tasks, the content and mix of which are determined by the state and are constantly changing. Even 'genericism' has not proved elastic enough to contain this for the strategic purposes of professionalization.

By the late 1970s loss of confidence in skills was being attributed to loss of specialization (DHSS 1978). Since then it has become clear that the definition, let alone the refinement, of relevant skills is difficult when departmental responsibilities are in constant flux. The same is, of course, true of the probation service, where the power of the state to force a change in methods by modifying the task has been vividly demonstrated (see Chapter 5). However, the probation service has the significant advantage over social services of being effectively a single-purpose agency. Many of the changes forced on it have not been welcome to staff, but the response has been relatively coherent and solidary.

Both Johnson (1972) and Halliday (1987) suggested that professionals working for state bureaucracies enjoy a kind of freedom derived from the assured supply of clients and the privacy of the classroom or social work interview. Under conditions of severe resource restrictions and centralization it is now obvious how contingent such autonomy really is. It is wholly unrelated to the concept of 'indeterminacy' elaborated by Jamous and Peloille (1970).

Local authorities have an array of responsibilities. In all of them the statutory base and thus procedures are constantly changing. In the context of declining resources the determination of priorities becomes the core problem. One response in many social services departments has been an unending cycle of reorganization and reallocation of posts. In many authorities the demands for new skills imposed by central government decision (of which child protection is the most dominating, but arguably community care the most radical departure) have been accompanied by local political commitment drastically to overhaul procedures and working practices within the frame of new thinking on equal opportunities.

If an effective nation-wide grouping of social workers were to have replaced the pre-Seebohm associations it would have had to happen immediately after reorganization in the 1970s. That was, however, the very era when the radical social work critique was most influential. Professionalism was cast as part of the reformist, consensual, therapeutic, paternal and controlling version of social work as reinserting clients into an unjust society. Trade unionism was seen by many to be both more authentic and more effective. Moreover, training was under the control, not of a professional association but of a quango with a chair and committee appointed by the Secretary of State. The profession's great and good have never dominated; in recent years the employer interest has been further strengthened.

If there ever was a window of opportunity for a unified professional lobby, it closed after 1979. Even if an agreed cognitive base had begun to form, a key part of the Thatcher government's agenda was the attack on professional monopolies; much more powerful occupations have been given the fearless brush-off. As a result, in the dominating local authority sector of social work, many individual workers have limited affiliation to wider groupings, in sharp contrast to NAPO in the probation service. BASW claims only about a third of social services department staff in membership; the number of active members must be tiny. As we have seen in the previous chapter, a very high premium is put on colleague support, but much of this is pitched 'at the feeling level'. Teams, offices and departments are inward-turned, the profession fragmented. Debates in the profession's own media are weakly developed: articles in *Community Care* and *Social Work Today* (now one journal) tend to the experiential and anecdotal; the *British Journal of Social Work* is written and read by educators and trainers, rather than by field practitioners.

Although possessing a recognized shared expertise does not guarantee the professional project, it is an irreducible necessity. The present institutional form of the biggest sector of social work employment and its ever more legalized and bureaucratized relationship with the state (Howe 1992; Parton 1991) make its development a receding possibility.

Clearly the professional project is not an unquestioned good, but, as we have seen from Chapter 1, the absence of an organized voice for the biggest sector of social work employment is a serious disadvantage in the clamour for media attention. Being part of a local authority and thus – rightly – being part of the political mechanisms of public accountability does not by itself stop parallel occupations having well-established representative bodies. Teaching, for example, has competing associations and thus several voices – but they are heard. Town planning has its Royal Institute. Both face very similar problems of political pressure and public controversy. Being a fertile news source, providing publicity material, having recognizable, reliable – and prefer- ably entertaining – 'experts' and talking heads are all essential. These activities do not guarantee media coverage, let alone approving treatment, and certainly not government sympathy – but their absence is undoubtedly a disadvantage, particularly when competing in this way is taken as a sign of fitness for purpose.

SOCIAL WORK AND GENDER

In a strictly numerical sense, social services work is indeed 'women's work'. A joint Department of Health/Social Services Inspectorate paper reports that, in 1990, 86.5 per cent of staff employed by social services departments in England and Wales were female. Over half the entire workforce was women working part-time in manual work, as home helps or care assistants. Among field social workers, who

> constitute about 10 percent of the total workforce . . . In 1988 74 per cent were female . . . At senior management level the situation is totally reversed. Seven out of eight Directors of Social Services in England and Wales are men and they make up 82 per cent of all senior managers . . . Forty-four of the 116 authorities in England and Wales have no women in the senior management teams and a further 39 have only one.

> (DoH/SSI 1991: 11, 5, 23)

When Etzioni (1969) identified what he claimed to be the new phenomenon of the 'semi-profession' he took a predominantly female workforce not only to be a common characteristic but as part of the explanation for the failure of teaching, nursing and social work (in the US) to achieve their professional aspirations. The solution, he suggests, is for such groups to accept their middle-ground status so as to avoid the 'dysfunctional consequences of trying to pass' because 'the normative principles and cultural values of the professions, organizations and female employment are not compatible' (Etzioni 1969: vii, vi). In their essay, Simpson and Simpson (1969) attribute the underdevelopment of such occupations to features of womanhood like being 'less attached to the principle of autonomy and less confident of their ability to claim or use it' and that 'they often share the general cultural norm that women should defer to men' (Simpson and Simpson 1969: 199). The authors are clearly not sanguine about this; they address issues of outright discrimination and describe the link between family responsibilities, discontinuous career, reduced aspirations and limited opportunity as a 'vicious circle' (Simpson and Simpson 1969: 229). The underlying explanation, however, fitting Etzioni's framework, is stubbornly idealist and reductionist: 'real professions' have genuine expertise; women are not in a position to acquire this, so those occupations where they predominate will fail to ascend the status ladder. Barred from the truly professional satisfaction of the 'exercise of skills', they will develop a 'holistic orientation', getting satisfaction from the response of the client. 'The act of service is its own reward, an expressive act, and it establishes a diffuse particularistic tie' (Simpson and Simpson 1969: 235–6). As is consistent with a functionalist perspective, the 'problem' for semi-professionals is socially constructed, and it is recognized that individual potential may be wasted. The ultimate legitimacy of the knowledge claims of real professionals and the naturalness of male occupancy of powerful positions remain, however, unquestioned because they inhere in a consensual social order.

As we have seen, more recent theorizing of the professions, whether neo-Marxist (Johnson 1972; Sarfatti Larson 1977) or neo-Weberian (Parkin 1979), has redefined the professionalizing process not as a passive state but as a continuing struggle. Knowledge is the key resource around which groups form to acquire, defend and extend 'operating space', deploying a range of weapons which will vary with market position and the possibility of either collegial or state-sponsored legal restrictions on practice. As Witz (1992) observes, until recently this debate has taken place quite separately from developing thinking on the gender division of labour in the home and in paid employment. Both Johnson (1972) and Parkin (1979) noted the simultaneous predominance of women in what Johnson called 'state mediated' professions, and the domination of more powerful 'collegial' groups by men, but did not consider the matter further. Hearn (1982), on the other hand, locates professionalism entirely within patriarchy: men predominate in those occupations which occupy important structural positions and have colonized the management of those (like social work and primary teaching) which deal with social reproduction.

Witz herself prefers a more multi-dimensional explanation, pointing out the pivotal significance that Sarfatti Larson (1977), Freidson (1986) and others attribute to the acquisition of formal credentials through higher education. The universities and the state are thus 'institutional sites for the mobilization of the means of professional closure' (Witz 1992: 65). During the nineteenth-century foundation of the bourgeois professions both the state and universities were exclusively male preserves. In the contemporary UK, despite right-on rhetoric and some cautious legislation and policy initiatives, the actuality is much the same: most of the powerful positions in the polity and in higher education are occupied by men. Perpetuating this virarchy may not itself be a purposeful enterprise, and yet the outcome is the continuing valorization of particular styles of thought, types of knowledge and personal qualities. For many in politics, the civil service and the universities, 'the right chap for the job' still looks reassuringly like oneself, public/civic life is more important than the private sphere, rationality superior to emotion, and hard science data and methods self-evidently closer to 'reality' than the soft knowledge of the humanities or social sciences. After all, where is their proof?

I do not, by this necessarily capsule characterization, intend to endorse either a wholly relative concept of knowledge and truth, or the school of thought that is confident that, if everyone was more like a woman, society's problems would be solved. An understanding of the media treatment and images of social work must, however, pay attention to its character as 'women's work' in a social order where to be female or to have female characteristics continues to be a source of disadvantage.

The devaluing of women's work is a complex triangle of the social construction of gender, the definition of skill, and the value put on caring. One outcome of feminist social science has been the challenging of the wholly androcentric assumptions embodied in standard models of social stratification and the scales used in its measurement (for a fuller discussion see Abbott and Sapsford (1987)). Most have been organized around the twin poles of 'real professions' like medicine and law and 'real work' like skilled trades. As the devastation of the industrial landscape in the 1980s opened up new perspectives, it has become much clearer how interlocked have been the ideas of 'skilled work', high rewards, and the exclusion of women from occupations. Technological change has revealed the force of questions like: what is the difference between an expert typist and a hot metal compositor? The answer is that the first is poorly paid, is thought to be semi-skilled and is a woman (unless he is a journalist, most of whom will proudly say they type with two fingers); the compositor used to be highly paid, was defined as skilled, and was always a man. Historic job definitions, patterns of recruitment and training (like lengthy apprenticeships), buttressed by male domination of management and unions, produced the artificial scarcity of the skilled worker, in ways wholly reminiscent of the production of the true professional. Thus it is not so much that women do semi-skilled work as that work is semi-skilled if women do it (Dex 1985).

Some manifestations of this process have been termed by Davies and Rosser the 'gendered job':

> ones which capitalise on the skills women have by virtue of having lived their lives as women. We emphasize that these skills go unacknowledged and unrewarded, that where they are seen at all they are seen as qualities which attach to a particular woman or women as a group.
>
> (Davies and Rosser 1986: 109)

Their research subjects were Higher Clerical Officers in the National Health Service, some of whom were employed in effect as office managers, with extensive responsibility: 'their immediate bosses, medical and paramedical staffs, used them to mediate the mysteries of policy, procedure and practice' (Davies and Rosser 1986: 104). The skills being used, but not paid for in terms of upgrading, were the 'priority-setting, scheduling, progress-chasing' management skills developed in running a home and family, the knowledge of the organization gained through continuity of employment, and the 'social skills crucial to the smooth running of the job' (Davies and Rosser 1986: 110). These were underpinned by the maturity, stability and local knowledge which also came with the package of older women with children of at least school age. As the authors are keen to emphasize (1986: 110), the consistent recruitment of women to these posts had merged the job and the qualities needed to the extent that the real skills they brought had disappeared, or rather were absorbed into the general attributes of a good employee, like honesty and courtesy. When one of their interviewees asked to go on a counselling course 'she was turned down. There was no desire, it seemed, to formalise her caring work, to see it as part of her job rather than as a quality of the person' (Davies and Rosser 1986: 103).

Where the job in question explicitly involves caring, the idea of distinctive knowledge or skill becomes even more blurred. Direct care-work will involve some combination of emotional labour and physical tending. As we have seen, there is at best ambivalence about the possibility or correctness of organized training in the management of emotions. Delta Airlines may put their staff through a rigorous pro-gramme (Russell Hochschild 1983), but social workers hesitate even to classify their ability to handle relationships as a learned skill in case it undermines authenticity, puts distance between them and the client – and perhaps implies that they do not have the intrinsic attributes of a good practitioner.

This reciprocal reluctance to reify and the undervaluing of emotional work may be explained by its frequent likening to friendship. The slippage between befriending, 'being friendly' and friendship is ever-present and a known problem in social work, and presumably in teaching and healthcare jobs too. Its use somehow rolls up informality, reciprocity, acceptance, approval and a holistic (or particularistic in an older jargon) orientation to the other person. People talk of friendship as somehow outside burdensome social conventions, but it is intensely rule-bound as Allan (1989) has demonstrated. We all know, but are deeply reluctant to admit, that such relationships occupy strict temporal, spatial and emotional territory. You get on fine with your neighbour as long as you keep off politics; have stimulating and amusing political discussions with your friend in the party branch but are glad there has never been a suggestion that you visit her home to endure her unruly children and eat her awful macrobiotic food. The direct result of this resistance to recognizing friendship as rule-bound is the impossibility of accepting the notion that it could involve learned skills. If it is not intuitive and spontaneous it is not genuine. In the world of paid employment, competencies that are not defined as having to be learned have little or no value, as Davies and Rosser (1986) underscore.

Essentially, then, a significant part of doing emotional work is seen as like doing friendship. It is natural and women are naturally better at it. Where emotional work goes beyond friendship it becomes analogous to what happens in the family. As Allan (1989) says, 'true friendship' is often distinguished by the use of kinship terminology: 'she is like a sister to me'. Within the family, emotional work is a crucial part of the process of social reproduction. Graham (1983), among many feminist writers, has argued that this is so much 'women's work' as to be constitutive of female identity. Women who reject it or do it badly are called upon to justify themselves. The 'reconstitution of the family on a daily basis' (Graham 1983: 23) also involves physical tending, particularly of young children, but also of the sick and frail elderly. Below the levels at which medical skills are thought to be required, the ability to carry this out is supposed to be the natural outcome of proper female predispositions and good socialization, with a little help from health visitors, clinics and popular child care manuals. Beyond that it should not have to be learned. To have to attend a family centre or be visited by a family aide is to be classified as deviant. Calls to increase the proportion of such knowledge in the school curriculum are an indicator of a supposed breakdown in the normal social order.

Thus, when women, particularly older women, take their accumulated experience of cooking, cleaning, co-ordinating, tending, and managing emotion into the workplace, it is not necessary to reward them highly. Anyone could do these things, as anyone could do those parts of field social work not governed by statute.

Social work, particularly in social services departments, is, then, saturated with gender issues. The lower-grade staff are mostly women not just because low-paid workers so often are, but also because of the nature of the work itself. So too are front-line social workers – and this tendency is again increasing after a brief spell when the recruitment of men rose in the early 1980s (DoH/SSI 1991). The most visible aspects of the work are thus done by women or by men in a woman's world. The senior management is persistently male, but operating over the very different terrain of local government bureaucracy and politics. This is the tabloid world of snoopers, bunglers, loony lefties and little Hitlers. Its combination with women claiming that 'doing what comes naturally' is actually difficult and demanding work makes for a considerable presentational problem.

PUBLIC ATTITUDES TO SOCIAL WORK

In 1989 *Community Care* (16 March) carried out a survey of social workers to compare their views of the perceived public standing of the profession with those in 1986 – a time, we have seen, of high anxiety. The 1989 survey showed that, among workers in children's homes, 69 per cent thought that public opinion of them had deteriorated, compared with 56 per cent for field workers and 55 per cent for other residential workers. Ninety-three per cent of the respondents who held this view blamed press coverage.

This feeling among practitioners, that social work operates in an inhospitable environment is, however, not new and not confined to the UK in the aftermath of child protection furores. Brawley, in the opening chapter of his how-to handbook for 'human services' workers in the US who wish to improve their public image, writes: 'For at least twenty years, social workers have agonized over their poor public image'. He assumes that the problem is that 'it is associated in the public mind with an unpopular field of endeavour – welfare' (Brawley 1983: 25). In the US to be a welfare client is to be dependent and is stigmatizing because of the 'deep-rooted tradition of the Protestant Ethic . . . with strong emphasis on individual responsibility and achievement' (Toren 1972: 148). The same position is taken by Golding and Middleton (1982) in *Images of Welfare*, which includes the first extended discussion of the media treatment of social work in the UK. Their central concern is the moral panic over supposed benefit scrounging in 1976. Although their quoted instances of hostile press coverage (1982: 89–91) relate to child deaths, Golding and Middleton's theme is that the antipathy of the right-wing newspapers to social work is rooted in social workers' central place in the 'nanny state', providing support for armies of workshy but shrewd 'undeserving poor'. 'Scroungerphobia' was part of a general realignment of attitudes towards a much more selective basis of entitlement to the benefits of the welfare state, lubricated by the resurrection of the centuries-old concept of the 'undeserving poor'.

One of the most interesting parts of Golding and Middleton's study is the discussion of journalists' own origins and attitudes to social welfare. Tellingly, though, no distinction is made by either authors or respondents between social work and social benefits. Yet in the UK, unlike many other countries, the delivery of social work and the social security system are administratively completely separate. Another section of Golding and Middleton's research reveals the extent to which, in the economic upheavals of the mid-1970s, the 'widespread antipathy to social security and to claimants reflected in the press clearly resonated with deep anxieties and indignation felt by many working class people' (Golding and Middleton 1982: 231).

But does the public also conflate social work and welfare benefits? Are social workers right to make a simple equivalence between negative media comment and adverse public attitudes? National opinion surveys commissioned by *Community Care* (5 March 1987) and *Social Work Today* (16 November 1989) appear to show a reasonably sympathetic public. The reports of both surveys express disappointment at the standing of the profession: 'Only one per cent of respondents place social workers in first place and only 15 per cent of all respondents placed them in the first three places' (*Community Care* 5 March 1987). In the *Social Work Today* survey

> only 13 per cent believe that social workers have a higher professional status than nurses ... only 14 per cent perceive social workers as having a higher status than teachers ... More than half the country believes that police officers have higher status than social workers.
>
> (*Social Work Today* 16 November 1989)

Social workers were ranked as having the same status as nurses by 42 per cent; as teachers by approximately half; and as police officers by 33 per cent. Doctors led the field. Overall, however, the journal accounts of the surveys treat the findings as encouraging. Respondents regarded social workers as doing difficult and necessary work. Between two-thirds and three-quarters of those questioned in all regions knew that they were employed by local authorities (*Community Care* 5 March 1987). This survey also reported widespread accurate knowledge of the range of social work tasks, despite relatively little first-hand contact.

> Most of the respondents had no recent, personal experience of dealing with the social services. One in five said they had had direct contact with social services or a social worker within the past two years. Not surprisingly the strata [*sic*] which had the most contact was the DEs, 29 per cent, compared to 19 per cent in the rest of the population.
>
> (*Social Work Today* 16 November 1989)

According to *Community Care*, when asked

> if they personally knew someone who had consulted or been visited by a social worker, 37 per cent replied affirmatively and there was only a marginal increase from older people (40 per cent of those over 55 replied in this way).
>
> (*Community Care* 5 March 1987)

The general interpretation of the data by the journals is resolutely upbeat. Golding, in his review of what is known of attitudes to social work, questions the justification for this 'cry of relief' (1991: 95). It would be better, he suggests, to understand the findings as support for the *idea* of social work. They do not necessarily indicate that the public has a favourable image of social workers themselves, if they are seen as effective, or whether social work services as now offered are what is needed. Finally: in 'Seeking to tap the affection of the public for care and caring, surveys have not ... baldly addressed the public's willingness to meet the cost of welfare in any sufficient depth' (Golding 1991: 96). That this is a complex issue was demonstrated by the 1992 UK general election when, despite widespread expressed concern for the quality of health and education services, alarming Conservative claims about the tax implications of Labour's spending plans seem to have attracted crucial support.

A question also remains as to the public's detailed appreciation of what social workers do and for whom. In the *Community Care* research (5 March 1987), 83 per cent of interviewees were aware that social workers undertake child supervision. But 54 per cent named 'assessment of welfare benefits'. As the survey says, 'While social workers *are* involved with welfare rights work, this . . . answer may indicate a confusion with the work of DHSS benefit offices.' This is doubly interesting: it could imply that an association with the benefit system does not have the negative effect that writers like Brawley (1983) and Golding and Middleton (1982) have assumed. On the other hand, it also suggests that public knowledge is very patchy. The list of possible tasks offered as a prompt to respondents to the *Community Care* survey contains some curiosities. Probation work is mentioned, but there is no indication as to whether the question of by whom probation officers are employed was pursued. Were they classified, inaccurately, under the 'local authority' heading? Nor is work with elderly people listed, although 'Dealing with mentally and physically handicapped people' is. The impact of this could be significant. It is hard to imagine (especially since probation work is included) that the survey made a fine distinction between field social workers and others working for social services departments. If not, then it must be probable that respondents' views of 'social work' embraced all the work of social services, including that done by both field social workers and – much valued – domiciliary services staff for elderly people. Rolling up this with the apparently uncontroversial nature of probation work as well could have had the effect of obscuring more disapproving attitudes specific to statutory social work with children and families.

Nevertheless, these limited data imply that, despite relatively low levels of the kind of first-hand or reliable second-hand knowledge that is suggested to be necessary for audiences to challenge media accounts (Philo 1990, and see Chapter 1), the public is (or was at the time of the surveys) remarkably unaffected by strident tabloid coverage. Perhaps, as people claim in other surveys, they get their actuality from broadcasting and qualify what they read in the national press with a clear understanding of editorial idiosyncrasies. Nevertheless, it would be unwise to conclude that social workers should be unconcerned with press coverage. The wider public may distinguish between press and broadcasting, but when media reactions are used as ammunition in the battle over the salience of an issue the distinction between the expressed attitude of a newspaper and the views of its audience tends to disappear. As Cohen (1973), Hall *et al.* (1978) and Schlesinger *et al.* (1991) demonstrate, the control culture uses the news media to talk to itself.

Chapter 9

Social work and the press: the prospects for peace

SOCIAL WORK IN THE PRESS: IS THERE A PROBLEM?

Social work is not the only occupation to maintain that it receives inordinately hostile press coverage and, by extension, to assume that it has a poor public image. Even such apparently unlikely groups as doctors (Karpf 1988) and the police force (Schlesinger *et al.* 1991) feel similarly aggrieved.

Unlike other occupations, though, the sense that social work is embattled extends beyond its members. At an everyday level, many non-social workers with whom I have discussed this project have exclaimed that social work 'of course' gets awful media treatment. Nearer the top of the hierarchy of credibility, the Kimberley Carlile inquiry panel took it for granted that news media treatment was a continuing background issue. Commenting on the coverage of the trial the report asserts that social workers 'by contemporary experience, are likely to be more than ordinarily castigated by a press that is often ill-motivated towards social work' and goes on to mention the 'bitter invective' (Carlile 1987: 9) in the (unnamed) *Daily Star*. The panel's 'Reasoned Decision' on holding its inquiry in private also refers to hostile 'selective press coverage' (Carlile 1987: 273).

The Butler Sloss report on the Cleveland events devotes a whole section to the news media (Cm 412 1988: 168–71). It opens: 'The media has [*sic*] played an important role in the Cleveland crisis at all stages.' After praising those who covered the inquiry for protecting the identities of the children, Butler Sloss comments on some news media behaviour. In terms of the customary ellipsis of legal talk this is a clear condemnation:

> In a highly charged Inquiry of great public interest and consequently newsworthy, we do not consider that the Chairman should have

powers to regulate the press . . . This lack of 'muscle' does, however, lay upon the media generally and editors in particular, the responsibility to observe moderation . . . Such a responsibility has not been recognised in certain quarters, and in this delicate and sensitive field where the welfare of children requires to be remembered, it was from time to time obviously overlooked.

(Cm 412 1988: 171)

One of the historic dictums of sociology is W.I. Thomas's assertion that, if social actors 'perceive situations as real, they are real in their consequences' (1932: 572). The real fear of the media portrayal of their actions is evident in ordinary social work discourse. The pain of individuals like Martin Ruddock and 'Social Worker 2', discussed in Chapter 7, is understood to be of enough shared relevance to appear in the academic/professional literature and trade press. Presumably the aim is to forewarn colleagues. Collectively, the ADSS has had a working party on the problem, and BASW (see Franklin and Parton 1991: *passim*) continues to struggle with increasing demands and shrinking resources. According to *Community Care* (26 September 1991) the general secretary has 'not just been called upon to explain his profession: he has been called upon to defend it' and has a 'right to feel battle-scarred'.

SO WHAT ARE THE DIMENSIONS OF THE PROBLEM?

The 'string of scandals, inquiries and consequent media attention' to which *Community Care* casually refers in the opening paragraph of its dissection of BASW's 'crisis' are not, in fact, about 'the profession': they all relate to local authority social services work with children and young people. Nor are 'the media' homogeneous. There are crucial cleavages along three dimensions: print/broadcast; broadsheet/tabloid market sector; local/national media.

Since the late 1980s a coincidence of events has focused attention on the financing of news media. Severe recession has drastically reduced potential advertising revenue. The post-Broadcasting Act 1990 franchise auction has mortgaged the income of most television companies for years to come. Meanwhile, the BBC is trying to package itself as suitably lean and hungry for the first renewal of its Charter in 1996.

Financial viability is clearly essential, no less for public-sector than for profit-driven media. Nevertheless, there are other organizational imperatives. Both the BBC and commercial broadcasting work within a statutory framework which requires their programming to be 'impartial'.

These demands were further strengthened for commercial television and radio under the 1990 Act. If social work organizations are tooled up to present their case, their scope for counteracting hostile editorializing will be even greater.

The majority of national daily newspapers are overtly Conservative, and yet this does not by itself dictate negative reporting of misadventure or even mistakes by social services. News will be framed by market niche almost as much as party politics. Thus the *Daily Telegraph* aims to provide abundant information in standard hard news format. The sheer volume of its crime and politics coverage ensures that a range of voices is presented. Despite the occasional reactionary bark in headline or editorial, the frame is one-nation Tory and can surprise with its sympathy. In contrast, *The Times* of the 1980s became an organ of the radical right, with an orientation to business and only erratic coverage of social issues.

For the *Guardian*, social policy and its political context are prime territory. The sneer that social workers are '*Guardian* readers' of course has a double significance: the paper is trying to capture highly lucrative job advertisements for all sectors of the caring business. As with its rival *The Independent*, the starting point will be receptiveness to professional dilemmas and claims to expert knowledge. Reciprocally with this, both non-Tory broadsheets can be comprehensive and scathing in their criticisms when professionals seem to have fallen short, as the coverage of the Rochdale events in the *Guardian* and of pin-down and similar practices in *The Independent* demonstrated.

The *Sun*, vulgar, strident, republican and anti-establishment, crudely patriotic, deeply conventional about gender, is the paper everyone loves to hate. Its shock value is the core of its appeal. When social workers get the full blast of its finely honed scorn of bureaucratic bunglers who manage to interfere with the dearly bought pleasures of working-class life and yet fail to stop the real deviants that threaten us, they are not specially privileged. The *Sun* is ideologically pro-individualism, anti-authority, and anti-state expenditure; it is not specifically anti-social work. Much the same applies to the *Daily Star* in its unfocused attempt to capture some of the same market.

Reading the *Daily Mirror* has always been more complex – in both an analytic and an everyday sense – as many of the case examples above have shown. Its continued support for Labour is an important commercial consideration, as well as a matter of principle. Albeit unevenly, its editorial line has, to date, tried to keep the value of the welfare state, of collective provision in general, and the idea of civil society in view. But it must also conform with popular 'common-sense' notions of traditional working-class family life and of the aetiology of social problems. It is also head-to-head with the *Sun*, which has had an impact upon the way news is framed. Continuing attempts to try and ground events in some kind of political and cultural context have tended to be overshadowed by the foreshortening demand for visual and textual drama and titillation, with their focus on concrete events and specific persons.

Sadly the *Mirror's* unique voice looks increasingly at risk. Since Robert Maxwell's death the paper has been treated by his creditors as one of the few recoverable assets and is being reshaped into a financial analyst's idea of a modern newspaper. It is hard to imagine that this will include pride in its socialist tradition.

Social workers should, however, comfort themselves that the mass tabloid attention span is short. Long trials, dense inquiry reports and convoluted policy issues will not be covered in detail, nor over a long period.

The most sustained adverse coverage of social work – even extending to probation and the voluntary sector – appears in the mid-market *Daily Mail* and, to a more limited extent, the *Daily Express*. The *Mail* is the paper most likely to pick up social work-related stories – unless they do not fit its paradigm, as with the Stephanie Fox inquiry report discussed in Chapter 2. Both it and the *Express* often supply 'background', not in the form of broadsheet-style semi-detached analysis, but highly opinionated pieces by right-wing commentators. Of all the national newspapers, the *Daily Mail* is the most pure in its support of individualist, *petit bourgeois*, patriarchal family values, as the case studies of social services work have shown and was also illustrated in its stance over the Cleveland child sex abuse events (Illsley 1989; Nava 1988; Parton 1991).

Few public employees escape the *Daily Mail's* suspicion. This is not because it is anti-state, but because of its advocacy of the Thatcherite 'strong state'. It trades on ontological and cultural insecurity. In its world the enemy is not so much within as everywhere: 'we' are pretty few; 'they' threaten to overwhelm. During my research it was even suggested to me that the *Daily Mail* has been unusual among Conservative papers in being critical of the police – for being too soft. The fracturing of the conventional separation of 'news' and 'comment' by the *Daily Mail's* passionate commitment to radical Toryism was manifest during the 1992 UK general election campaign – and the subject of a number of sanctimonious articles in other newspapers! It once had the slogan that the *Daily Mail* was for 'busy thinkers'. The aim then and now seems to be to supply ready-made opinions: these do not favour state social work.

Today serves as an index of the profound changes in the newspaper industry over the last decade. During the early 1990s it began to settle into a non-Tory magazine-style paper for younger family readers. The pitch is of a down-market consumerist *Independent*, not intrinsically hostile to welfare institutions.

The same market considerations that govern the treatment of social work by the national press apply to local media, but with a different outcome. Party political alignment and criticisms of individuals must be kept in check to avoid alienating both potential readers and politicians and functionaries. Local journalists rely upon the goodwill of their contacts. Among the readers will be actors in the dramas reported. Those in their social network will be able to repudiate inaccurate accounts, with potentially damaging commercial consequences. Subjectively, media exposure close to home must be particularly unpleasant for social workers, but objectively the tone and content will usually be very different from national press coverage, as material from local papers in Oldham (Chapter 2), Leicester (Chapter 3), Nottingham (Chapters 4 and 7) and the west country (Chapter 5) have shown. Essentially the national press takes few risks when it delivers extravagant personal attacks, and partial, oversimplified – or straightforwardly inaccurate – reporting of complex social issues. Local media have a lot to lose.

It is also clear that the condemnatory and sometimes vicious newspaper criticism that has lodged in social work's folk memory relates mainly to three clusters of events: a small number of criminal trials around 1985; the Cleveland events of 1987–8; and the Rochdale/Orkney satanic abuse controversies from 1990. All these related to social services work with children. Other local authority responsibilities like the care of elderly people, far from being the target of criticism, often pass unreported. If they become news they are fitted into another framework, for example, politics or social policy.

Local authority departments sometimes get positive coverage, in the national as well as the local press. The reporting of their involvement in counselling those caught up in disasters was analysed in Chapter 7. Neither this, nor the seeming tacit acceptance of social services' work with elderly people is straightforwardly reassuring, though. As we have seen in Chapter 4, news media ignore the concerns of elderly people because of their peripheral social and economic status. Conversely, the approval of griefwork follows from its consonance with conservative notions of individualism and deservingness.

The probation service, formerly almost invisible in the news media, has been forced to enter the image-building business. Its effectiveness has, predictably, been greatest with the local media and the liberal broadsheets. Again only limited comfort can be drawn from positive media treatment, as the publicity drive is a direct consequence of the government's agenda of more punitive community disposals. Whether bodies like NAPO can, having gained media attention, use it to pursue the more radical parts of their agenda remains to be seen.

Most voluntary organizations have a complex symbiotic relationship with the news media, in which campaigns on issues, the maintenance of public visibility, revenue-raising, the establishment of humanitarian credentials, and stereotyped emotional responses are densely interwoven. In their different styles, most newspapers respond to voluntary sector social work activity, but this imposes its own constraints. Even social work with children will be criticized if, as in the case of ChildLine (Chapter 7), conventional family authority is challenged. Nor may the populist style needed for very large-scale fund-raising mesh easily with progressive ideas about gender roles and domestic violence.

Are we then to conclude that social work only gets intense national press coverage when the issue involves some combination of violent crime, unlawful sexual behaviour, sentimentalized 'tragic tots', or alleged professional/bureaucratic failure? Such scenarios undoubtedly fulfil all the editorial and newsgathering requirements of newspapers in every sector of the market, as the case studies abundantly demonstrate. Readers of *The Independent* can be outraged and fascinated by pin-down, of the *Daily Mail* by the parents' protestations in Rochdale, of the *Sun* by the vivid horror of Tyra Henry's death.

Describing what *does* get reported is interesting, but for an understanding of the press coverage of social work, investigating what *does not* make the news is more significant. Thus in 1985, shortly after the intense media exposure of the Tyra Henry case, a trial (Reuben Carthy) in Nottingham involving allegations about social services and with a racial dimension was virtually ignored. Another 1985 case with plenty of sordid 'human interest' details in Oldham (Charlene Salt) was widely reported but was treated in isolation. It was not mapped on to the larger paradigm of state social work failure, neither were later cases in London (Stephanie Fox and Sudio Rouse).

Social workers' bewilderment at press hostility is intensified by what are said to be contradictory accusations: over Tyra Henry intervention was insufficient; in Rochdale there was too much. (The fact that Mr Justice Douglas Brown finally ruled that there was no evidence of ritual abuse is immaterial. Many newspapers had condemned Rochdale Social Services as mistaken months beforehand.)

Beneath this apparent arbitrariness over when and how social services work is criticized, however, lies a deeper consistency. What is at stake, as we have seen in Chapters 2, 3 and 8, is the struggle to define the boundary of the 'normal family' and the corresponding legitimacy of state supervision of the private domestic behaviour of those who fall outside it. This long-running struggle to identify the 'dangerous' minority has spawned a complex two-stage process to which aspects of moral panic theory can usefully be applied (Cohen 1973, 1985; Hall *et al.* 1978; Parton 1985; 1991; and see Chapter 1).

The first stage focused on the mid-1980s cluster of very highly publicized trials and inquiries, following the deaths of children in London. Politicians and professionals cried 'How could this happen?' A scenario was developed in which children coming to harm was explained by the lack of rigorous training and an incapacity to act decisively on the part of professional staff, combined with local councillors' preoccupation with a brew of municipal socialism and the politics of race.

The solutions proposed were to make training more scientific and legalistic; tighten up the legislative framework; catalogue those needing control; and be ready to throw the book at them. Both Cohen and Hall *et al.*, despite their different theoretical fundament, model this 'reaction' phase of the moral panic in terms of a coincidence of interest in the control culture over what action should be taken – even if motivations differ, as Cohen (1985) has since observed. Legislators, the judiciary, professionals and pressure groups harmonize together through the news media in a chorus of mutual reinforcement. Further confirmation of the correctness of their concern will be provided by the reporting of every remotely related issue in those media through the 'sensitization' process.

The search for the infallible practitioner and dangerous family has been less coherent. What we have witnessed is, arguably, a new manifestation of this reaction phase. Instead of another circuit of the same panic, the issue spun away like a satellite leaving its orbit, to be recaptured in another public outcry.

By the 1980s a number of developments, including that breakup of the liberal establishment so desired by the Thatcherite right, had made the social construction of social problems a much more fragmented and unpredictable process. In this post-modern policy-making arena the players were more numerous and less controllable. Many were competing with each other for resources (Schlesinger *et al.* 1991). Not all those professionally involved in the surveillance of the family shared the government's fiscal interest in restricting the size of the class of deviants. On the contrary: voluntary agencies had to expand their brief to sustain and increase funding; peripatetic consultants (many of them former local authority social workers) had proliferated at the same time as in-house social services training was being run-down through expenditure restrictions. Despite the popular appeal of neo-liberal individualism, among professionals a new version of the conventional patriarchal family, as systematically oppressive and frequently violent, had begun to permeate everyday practice wisdom.

Suddenly social workers were exposed not only to the notion of widespread physical abuse of children, but to apparently authoritative individuals and groups convinced that 'normal' sexual abuse was endemic. It was also being asserted that the existence of ritual abuse would inevitably be established once institutional resistance from the police and others was overcome. Having been excoriated for failing to intervene, the best course for management and front-line staff would surely be to act on any suspicion. This was the logical failsafe strategy.

Some commentators have suggested that press coverage of the social workers at the centre of the child death moral panics placed them in the role of 'folk devil'. The evidence does not sustain this interpretation. Being the lead in the moral drama means taking action; social workers were usually accused of culpable inaction. Even at their most harsh, the press reserved tags like 'animal', 'monster', 'brute' and 'evil' for the offenders themselves (see Chapters 2 and 3).

Whatever the actuality, the symbolic importance of the Cleveland events was that they raised the possibility that child sex abuse is not exceptional, but pervasive. This spectre of widespread unlawful behaviour reversed the characteristics of the signification spiral (Hall *et al.* 1978) described in Chapter 1. Instead of the reclassification of a minority as beyond the legality threshold by criminalizing their behaviour, the social location of the boundary of social conformity was being challenged. As the class of dangerous families threatened to become morally and practically uncontainable, the second-stage panic developed, in which the 'problem' was not abusive parents but ill-judged interference in private family life. Social workers now more nearly fitted the 'folk devil' description. Among the 'inventory' of their characteristics were dogmatic feminism; gullibility; impetuousness; pathological secretiveness; lack of factual knowledge and of basic techniques, for example conducting an evidentially reliable interview; and a tendency to useless dramatic gestures like dawn raids.

This second-stage panic quickly went around three sub-circuits. An nth-level simplification of the meaning of the Cleveland events was applied in Rochdale, apparently verified by the subsequent court judgement (see Parton 1991 and Chapter 3) and also used to frame media presentation of the long-drawn-out Orkneys episode. The impact on the public seemed to be real enough. Declining reports about suspected abuse resulted in an NSPCC campaign to reassure the public (see Chapter 7).

This would seem to be an important datum on media effect, an issue central to any evaluation of whether social work has a substantial and distinctive problem with its media coverage. One assertion can be made with confidence: the intense coverage of an issue in the news media does not constitute evidence of prior public concern, even though it is often to the mutual benefit of media organizations and members of the control culture to assert that it does. Calling this process 'legislation by tabloid' (Franklin and Parton 1991: 29) could imply the application of a pluralist concept of news media autonomy (see Ericson *et al.* 1987 and Chapter 1). The reality is that most of the commercial press is easily mobilized to defend the status quo, especially by Conservative governments: 'legislation *via* tabloid'.

It is not necessary to subscribe to a class analysis to see that what appears in the national press is the relatively powerful talking to each other, whether one calls it the control culture or the policy community (Schlesinger *et al.* 1991, quoting Kingdon 1984). Of course the aim can be to create public concern, as the Hall *et al.* (1978) account of the moral panic argues. Where the audience has no other basis on which to make a judgement – about *Salmonella* in chicken flocks for example (Fowler 1991) – media messages are likely to be powerful (Philo 1990).

As we have seen in Chapter 1, media effects research remains sectarian and very disputatious. Active agnosticism would seem to be the best stance. To assume that the effect is nil risks allowing the agenda of the powerful to go unchallenged; to theorize media messages as completely determining audience understanding of the issue in question is disempowering and patronizing. Few social workers (or academics) conceive themselves as other than highly sophisticated consumers of media output, able to apply a critical reading equally to the soap opera, the Brecht play, the women's magazine, the television documentary, and the copy of the *Sun* in the coffee room. Applying this to consumers as a whole is a useful corrective against crudely mechanistic or conspiratorial accounts of news media functioning.

DOES SOCIAL WORK TAKE ITS PRESS TOO SERIOUSLY?

As an occupation, social work is unusually badly placed to handle a hostile press. Local authority social services, the target for most attack, are in the least advantageous position of all.

Social work professional culture has maintained 'use of self' in the foreground. Originally derived from the psychodynamic tradition, one-to-one relationship skill, as we have seen in Chapters 7 and 8, is the core expertise on which everyone from harassed front-line workers (DHSS 1978) to the Barclay Committee (NISW 1982) can agree. It has provided an important practical and symbolic focus throughout the long uncertainties of the Seebohm-inspired restructuring of the 1970s (Cmnd 3703 1968; DHSS 1978) and the more fundamental realignments of the 1980s (Johnson 1990; Wilding 1992).

Contemporary one-to-one skills in social work are eclectic; the epistemological individualism of psychodynamic models has been largely rejected. Occupational culture remains, however, infused with reductionist assumptions which have been bolstered by the influx of US-generated self-help therapies and the medicalization of child protection. Social workers have persistent difficulties with social structural explanations. This discomfort can even coexist with a strong visceral commitment to feminism and to fighting other kinds of systemic inequality. In respect of the news media this helps to explain why the fulminations of the tabloid press are too easily interpreted as specific people, who should know better, personally attacking people who did their best, instead of the collision of two institutions operating in a capitalist socio-economic framework. (And the corollary: that, if individual journalists were better informed, the coverage would be more understanding.)

Those for whom the self is the tool makes themselves vulnerable, but many can ground their performance in some criteria of success. For actors there is the critical reception and behinds on seats, students' response for teachers. Social workers have no such point of reference and perhaps cannot hope for it. Social 'health' is ideological; even voluntary clients should not be expected to be 'grateful'; many clients are the subjects of involuntary statutory control. Will the state or the public say 'good work', and on what possible basis?

Unable to justify what they do by the output, social workers are driven back on to their input. Even here there is little refuge given the lack of consensus over cognitive base and technique (see Chapter 8). Social workers cannot console themselves in the way that a surgeon might – that, although the patient died, the procedure was technically brilliant. Worse, the continuing focus on one-to-one competency and personal attributes (DHSS 1978; England 1986; Holme and Maizels 1978) works away from the refinement of knowledge and skills. Authenticity of feeling is constantly stressed; professional concern is sometimes confused with friendship. The deliberate use of theoretical approaches is characterized as imposing distance between worker and client. Social workers are thus left metaphorically naked, asking to be judged as persons and by their good intentions – while most occupations are praised or blamed for their results.

Faced with a client in this kind of dilemma, a social worker might well recommend a self-help group. Many social work teams seem to function in this way. Naturally they tend to focus on experiential exchange and mutual emotional support. More formal professional development and campaigning should be undertaken by the employer and the trade union/professional association. Yet neither of the latter seems to provide consistent support and protection.

To what extent front-line practitioners should be expected to take full responsibility for their actions seems to be ambiguous. The Kimberley Carlile inquiry panel commented that social workers 'must be treated as public servants whose skills and judgements are subject to the dictates of public employers' (Carlile 1987: 275). One dimension of the Tyra Henry controversy (Chapter 2) was Lambeth councillors' assertion of their right to control details of practice (specifically racial considerations in child protection work). This statutory right was subsequently endorsed by the inquiry report (Henry 1987). The logical extension of this, for all authorities, is that councillors' responsibility includes protecting their junior staff from having to deal directly with adverse publicity, unless and until any internal disciplinary procedures are properly completed. Despite this, when a department's practice is criticized, many practitioners seem to feel that they cannot expect their own managers, let alone the elected members, to give them the protection which their public servant locus entitles them (for example Ruddock 1991; Tonkin in *Community Care* 5 March 1987).

Should not the trade union/professional association fill this vacuum? This remains highly problematic. BASW is not a trade union. Local authority social work staff wishing to protect both their conditions of service and professional concerns are faced with the necessity of having to join both NALGO and BASW, with all that implies financially and in terms of commitment if one wishes to be an active member. Presumably this cash problem, coupled with the territorial and cognitive frag-mentation of the profession (see Chapter 8), explains BASW's having only about a third of social services staff in membership (*Community Care* 26 September 1991), while 80 per cent of local authority staff up to area management level belong to NALGO (significantly higher than the overall membership of about 70 per cent of staff). As a result, BASW is not well placed, either in terms of resources or credibility, to position itself as a powerful voice for non-probation social work.

CAN SOCIAL WORK LEARN TO LIVE WITH ITS PRESS OR EVEN IMPROVE IT?

Press criticism of social work, and specifically local authority social services work, is not going to go away. On the contrary, the dismemberment of local authority education responsibilities and the residualization of council housing will leave social services as the biggest spending department, whatever the structure of local government. It is likely, therefore, to be under yet more scrutiny from local media and to have a high profile when national government policy and spending strategy are in the news.

In terms of electoral accountability this should be welcome. Large swathes of social expenditure have passed from direct central and local government control to bodies like housing associations, arm's-length quangos, and large charities. While they can appear informal and user-friendly, in reality many of these are undemocratic and impenetrable to users, to the local electorate, and even parliament.

Developments in the news media are unlikely to produce a Pauline conversion to the cause of state-provided welfare. Those that are already commercial will remain ruthlessly profit-driven; those that have public service responsibilities are also facing cash problems. Even if the Tory national press shifts to support of a more corporate style of capitalism, the priority is likely to be those sectors which feed private consumption, industry and commerce in a more direct and transparent way: health, housing, transport, energy, education and training. The needs of marginal families, elderly people, and people with mental and physical difficulties will remain secondary.

Newspapers' dependence on advertising revenue also ensures that they will have a continuing stake in the family household as a vital unit of consumption. There is a material as well as an ideological motive behind the promotion of traditional family structures and a conventional gender division of labour by, for example, the *Daily Mail*.

It is equally unlikely that the orientation of newsgathering routines to the institutional order will shift. The news agenda will remain dominated by the definitions of the government of the day, by the other sections of the polity, and by financial and business institutions. Judicial and medical frames of reference will be treated as definitive in preference to a professional social work interpretation. The mass tabloids will continue to cultivate their police rather than their social services contacts. Explanations will still be framed in terms of bunglers and monsters rather than inadequate investment or the violence inscribed in conventional masculinity.

The Broadcasting Act 1990 was a quintessentially Thatcherite statute. Promising deregulation and 'a light touch' the new regime for commercial broadcasting involves more detailed, centrally imposed control than its predecessor. A positive aspect of this is that documentary-style programmes must still be screened, subject to the tighter demands for impartiality also enshrined in the Act. The bad news is that these need no longer be shown in peak time and are likely to be starved of resources. As the new franchises took effect in January 1993, media commentators gloomily grumbled about 'tabloid TV' in news and current affairs, meaning a shift to the same preoccupations with people and events, rather than complex causes or processes. This does not augur well for social work and social welfare, which can so easily be simplified, personalized and sensationalized.

One of the recurring themes of this study has been the different orientation of local media. The local press stood up to the late 1980s recession better than many other sectors of the news media. This demand for local news, coupled with its relative cheapness, may produce more local programming on television but warnings of trivialization abound. A *Guardian* critic was not impressed by the first few days of Meridian (the new franchise holder for the English south coast region), saying of the early evening news:

> Most of it is drivel, the worst kind of junk telly . . . looking for what is known in the trade as 'Ooh-just-fancy-that stories' [including] the eight-year-old girl who was rescued from a fire by the ghost of her great grandfather (reported as fact); and a ferret's funeral.
>
> (*Guardian* 7 January 1993)

Over the last twenty years, the social work profession's response to its perceived bad press has been uncritical pained incomprehension, and often passivity – even when indignant. The goal of an entirely 'good press' is unrealistic and potentially frustrating. Nevertheless, some positive coverage and a more perceptive, robust, and resilient reaction to negative news treatment are achievable. What should be the components of such a strategy?

Put the problem in perspective

- The problem must be put in perspective. Much is said about 'risk' in social work. Local authority workers are permanently 'at risk' of hostile news media coverage, not only when something goes wrong – they may well be treated unsympathetically when there is no failure in the delivery of service. But the risk attaches only to some kinds of work with some kinds of clients, and even then raucous tabloid treatment is not inevitable. In part 'a bad press' is the structural outcome of the complex and contested nature of the social work task and the political ideology of some national newspapers. Much personal and corporate wear-and-tear could be saved by acceptance of this, alongside clear plans for its containment.

Develop media education for social workers

Both individual professionals and representative bodies need media education. Understanding news production as a commercially driven industry, and having a basic grasp of how it works, would forestall the waste of resources on attempts to make links with or 'enlighten' media that are unlikely ever to endorse state welfare. Social workers know that they have their own jargon and ideology – and that daily reality often falls short of their claims. Appreciating the parallel myths and aspirations of the journalists' world – rugged individualist reporters; brave campaigning editors telling the proprietor to get lost; the autonomy of media organizations from both their audience and the socio-political base – would dispose of the unhelpful notion of the media/source encounter as between two rational free agents in search of truth.

Such an awareness should form part of basic training, should be a regular element of in-service training, and should also be provided by the professional and trade union bodies. Nor should this be instrumental 'how-to' tips and hints limited to the staff likely to have to handle media relations. Putting news media within a proper conceptual framework should help to dispel collective fantasies and anxieties, which means addressing all members of the organization.

In December 1992 CCETSW received a '"fairly robust"' letter from the minister about the contemporary relevance of its training guidelines (*Guardian* 13 December 1992). This would seem an apposite moment to redraw the DipSW competencies to take explicit account of the demands of social work as particularly intense emotional work. Neglect of this has been persistent, perverse and astonishing. Becoming less fearful of the news media should form a small but crucial part of addressing the problem.

Take media reactions seriously

Social services departments must take media relations as seriously as do voluntary sector organizations and the probation service. This will not be easy. Local authorities are formally accountable to the public through the electoral process. Elected members have their own interests to pursue where both local and national media are concerned, and may or may not be willing for professional staff to deal directly with news organizations. Government legislation requires any local authority publicity to be non-party-political. Individual cases will raise complex issues of client confidentiality and there may be legal restrictions on identifying participants. Media relations policies are expensive in staff costs; they can be portrayed as a diversion of resources from direct work with clients.

All this said, however, a policy based on responding 'no comment' to nearly all requests for information or reaction is now wholly inadequate. As Schlesinger et al. (1991) illustrate in their study of the criminal justice system, gaining publicity is now an essential part of the struggle to maintain or enlarge your share of declining state funds. This is not merely a haphazard fall-out of the crisis of state expenditure: image-making is one of the 'disciplines' that has been imposed on public sector organizations as part of the Conservative government's drive to create quasi-markets (Hudson 1992).

Of course if hospitals, universities, the probation service and the rest really were businesses in a market-place, they would have a very different degree of control over what they produce (and cease to produce), at what price, by what technology, and for which intended customers. Behind the righteous talk of freedom, choice and the minimal state is an actuality of tight – and increasing – central control (Shaw 1993). In the absence of real market criteria, the surface trappings of being 'business'-like are demanded as a surrogate. (For most staff the material base of 'an attractive remuneration package' comparable with the private sector is noticeably absent.) However uncongenial, social work organizations and local authority departments will have to join in this contest in representation or further increase their market disadvantage.

There is no doubt that for social work these disadvantages are going to be unusually hard to shift. Social services departments can only create relationships with news media within the remit and resources allowed by the elected members in respect of the whole authority. The aggregate of these legitimate restrictions will inevitably hobble the ADSS, as a potential voice of professional social work, even if directors were not in the unenviable position of administering central government directives and local cuts.

BASW is similarly in a very weak structural position: not only does minority membership deny it the resources and standing to be an effective pressure group, but professional education and licensing is in the hands of CCETSW, a government-appointed and increasingly employer-dominated quango. Given the indirect government control over the cognitive base of social work through its determination of social services' responsibilities (see Chapter 8), constructing a more unified and powerful professional lobby, whether based on BASW or not, will be difficult.

Trade union membership is vital to workplace relations, but NALGO (now part of Unison) or an equivalent cannot serve as a lobby about, for example, the details of proposed legislation on mental health. If non-probation social workers want to see the emergence of a highly visible 'authorized knower' for their job and its manifold problems, they will have to reconsider their distaste for 'professionalization'. What configuration and commitment of effort is needed to try to gain greater public visibility? It will certainly not come about by magic.

If the debate on social work as a 'profession' were reopened in a more pragmatic and bottom-up style, how should the gender dimension of the occupation be understood? Whatever professional control amounts to, its achievement is a struggle. Social work has made little headway so far. As I hope that Chapter 8 has shown, it is a profound misunderstanding to attribute this directly to the high proportion of women in front-line social work. Certainly it is 'women's work', so women are both drawn and driven into it. It is women's work because it is related to the control and support of the family, the principal site of 'caring' and social reproduction. These activities, although central to the capitalist economy and thus politically highly sensitive, are nevertheless undervalued. 'Femininity' is so constructed that being skilled in doing them comes naturally, so need not be rewarded in the market-place.

Higher priority for social work and its clients will come not by masculinizing the profession but by socio-political changes in family and gender relations. In the mean time, less emphasis on intuition and common sense in occupational culture would strengthen the assertion that emotional labour is real work requiring distinctive learned skills.

Develop media relations strategies

Social work lobbies and service providers need simultaneous reactive and pro-active media relations strategies. Both are clearly illustrated in the scrutiny of the probation service and the voluntary sector in Chapters 5 and 6. Reaction is not only 'damage limitation', but also the willingness to be the source of clear, accurate and plentiful background information to newsgatherers, often about issues which do not affect the organization or department directly, as when a local paper wants to cover a national controversy. Much of this input will not be attributed or even be easily visible. It is a long-term investment in media personnel's background knowledge and goodwill.

If the organization becomes newsworthy, some concrete response to media approaches should always be available, even where the situation is recent, confusing and rapidly changing. Even a ringing declaration that 'everything possible will be done' has utility, as the Wirral case (Chapter 4) illustrates. An absence of reaction will produce a vacuum which will assuredly be filled by more highly motivated or better organized sources: aggrieved relatives, pressure groups, local politicians, doctors, the police, etc. Media-literate voluntary organizations (Chapter 6) and those social services departments that have adopted an active strategy, like Bradford (Walder 1991) and County Cleveland (Treacher in *Local Government Chronicle* 27 July 1988), all stress that coherence and consistency is vital. A limited number of staff should deal with the media and they should develop and stick to a unified policy line. Internal conflict in any organization is dramatic and very accessible news, as the Tyra Henry case (in Chapter 2) and the Nottinghamshire elderly persons' homes saga (in Chapter 4) both illustrated. Honesty and accountability do not entail conducting all your disputes in public.

Whatever the perception of constant vulnerability, the current reality is that most social services departments rarely appear in the news media, even locally. This is not good news. If media messages have any impact at all, the implication is that what most people will know of social services is accumulated fragments about real or alleged failures, disputes and scandals. Social services must try systematically to feature in the news when things go right as well as when they are wrong. If NACRO clients, with appropriate safeguards, are willing to take part in giving work with offenders actuality, why not those of social services? Departments' work consists almost entirely of human drama and 'triumph over tragedy'. The national mid-market tabloids are probably a lost cause (except *Today*), but even the mass tabloids might respond occasionally to well-set-up material aligned to national issues like the successful placing of older children with adoptive families, or social services-inspired self-help groups, or successful examples of elderly people supporting themselves in their own homes. Conversely, new issues of concern like the demands on elderly carers might provide a superficially non-political platform for some tabloid campaigning.

Local media remain, however, the obvious target for publicity efforts not only by individual local authorities, but by national lobbies too. Local paid-for and free newspapers penetrate deep into the consciousness of an area. They are accessible; often eager for copy (especially in the case of free papers and local radio); their news values encompass 'good' and relatively unexciting news; and it is in their commercial interest not to be simplistic or overly partisan on local issues (see the fuller sections on local papers in Chapters 4, 5 and 6). If active cultivation of news media contacts can result in a probation officer's promotion to senior probation officer passing the threshold into news (see Chapter 5), the wealth of potential material provided by a day in the life of social services is obvious.

Television may begin to open up too, although the size of even the smaller franchise regions will inhibit both the intensity of viewer identification and the cultivation of strong relationships with newsgatherers. Developing cogent, authoritative, stylish and telegenic 'talking heads' should still form an important element in social services' media relations work.

It may be seem a profound contradiction that a directly elected, publicly funded body should have to seek a second legitimation for its activities by a direct appeal to the populace through the news media – but it is the new reality. Most other similar social formations have entered the arena with more or less enthusiasm. Threatened teaching hospitals employ public relations consultants; universities acquire logos and press officers. For many voluntary organizations to lose their public profile would be to cease to exist: defining their mission, direct work, public education, campaigning for policy change, lobbying, appealing for funds, and cultivating their relations with the news media are so closely bound together as to be seamless. The probation service is rapidly – if with un-even effectiveness – developing its news management skills. Social services work must overcome attitudinal and institutional barriers and enter the public profile tournament. The prize is certainly not unsolicited press eulogies of social work, nor even the gentler handling by reporters and their editors of practitioners or departments involved in public controversy. The real stakes are bigger still: defending the public mandate and resources required to meet the needs and defend the rights of some of our most vulnerable fellow citizens.

Bibliography

Abbott, P. and Sapsford, R. (1987) *Women and Social Class*, London: Tavistock.

Aldridge, M. (1990) 'Social work and the news media – a hopeless case?' *British Journal of Social Work*, 20, 6: 611–20.

Aldridge, M. and Hewitt, N (eds) (1994) *Confronting Broadcasting: Access Policy and Practice in North America and Europe*, Manchester: Manchester University Press.

Allan, G. (1989) *Friendship*, Hemel Hempstead, Herts.: Harvester Wheatsheaf.

Bamford, T. (1990) *The Future of Social Work*, London: Macmillan.

Becker, H. (1967) 'Whose side are we on?' *Social Problems*, 14: 239–47.

Bevins, A. (1990) 'The crippling of the scribes', *British Journalism Review*, 1, 2: 13–17.

Bolger, S., Corrigan, P., Docking, J. and Frost, N. (1981) *Towards Socialist Welfare Work*, London: Macmillan.

Boyd, A. (1990) *Broadcast Journalism* (revised edition), Oxford: Heinemann.

Brawley, E. (1983) *Mass Media and Human Services: Getting the Message Across*, Beverley Hills, Calif.: Sage.

Brewer, C. and Lait, J. (1980) *Can Social Work Survive?* London: Maurice Temple Smith.

Carlile (1987) *A Child in Mind; Protection of Children in a Responsible Society: the Report of the Commission of Inquiry into the Circumstances Surrounding the Death of Kimberley Carlile*, London: London Borough of Greenwich.

Central Council for Education and Training in Social Work (CCETSW) (1991) 'Rules and Requirements for the Diploma in Social Work', *CCETSW Paper 30* (second edition), London: CCETSW.

Chibnall, S. (1977) *Law and Order News*, London: Tavistock.

ChildLine (1992) *Annual Report 1992*, London: ChildLine.

Chippindale, P. and Horrie, C. (1990) *Stick It Up Your Punter: the Rise and Fall of the Sun*, London: Hutchinson.

Cm 412 (1988) *Report of the Inquiry into Child Abuse in Cleveland 1987*, London: HMSO.

Cm 424 (1988) *Punishment, Custody and the Community*, London: HMSO.

Cm 849 (1989) *Caring for People*, London: HMSO.

Cm 965 (1990) *Crime, Justice and Protecting the Public*, London: HMSO.

Cm 966 (1990) *Supervision and Punishment in the Community*, London: HMSO.

Cm 1102 (1990) *Report of the Committee on Privacy and Related Matters* (the Calcutt Report), London: HMSO.

Cm 2135 (1993) *Review of Press Regulation*, London: HMSO.

Cmnd 3703 (1968) *Report of the Committee on Local Authority and Allied Personal Social Services* (the Seebohm Report), London: HMSO.

Cohen, S. (1973) *Folk Devils and Moral Panics: the Creation of the Mods and Rockers*, London: Paladin (first published 1972, London: McGibbon and Kee, now in third revised edition 1987, Oxford: Basil Blackwell).

—— (1985) *Visions of Social Control*, Oxford: Polity Press with Basil Blackwell.

Cohen, S. and Young, J. (eds) (1981) *The Manufacture of News: Deviance, Social Problems and the Mass Media* (revised second edition), London: Constable.

Corrigan, P. and Leonard, P. (1978) *Social Work Practice Under Capitalism*, London: Macmillan.

Coulshed, V. (1991) *Social Work Practice: an Introduction* (second edition), London: Macmillan.

Counter Information Services/Community Development Project (CIS/CDP) (1975) *Cutting the Welfare State (Who Profits?)*, London: CIS/CDP Information Unit.

Cumberbatch, G. and Negrine, R. (1992) *Images of Disability on Television*, London: Routledge.

Curran, J. and Seaton, J. (1991) *Responsibility Without Power: the Press and Broadcasting in Britain* (fourth edition), London: Routledge.

Dant, T. and Johnson, M. (1991) 'Growing old in the eyes of the media', in B. Franklin and N. Parton (eds) *Social Work, the Media and Public Relations*, London: Routledge.

Davies, C. and Rosser, J. (1986) 'Gendered jobs in the health service: a problem for labour process analysis', in D. Knight and H. Willmott (eds) *Gender and the Labour Process*, Aldershot, Hants.: Gower.

Davies, M. (1981) *The Essential Social Worker: a Guide to Positive Practice*, London: Heinemann.

Department of Health and Social Security (DHSS) (1978) *Social Service Teams: the Practitioners' View*, London: HMSO.

Department of Health/Social Services Inspectorate (DoH/SSI) (1991) *Women in Social Services: a Neglected Resource*, London: HMSO.

Dex, S. (1985) *The Sexual Division of Work*, Hemel Hempstead, Herts.: Harvester Wheatsheaf.

Dingwall, R. (1989) 'Some problems about predicting child abuse and neglect', in O. Stevenson (ed.) *Child Abuse: Public Policy and Professional Practice*, Hemel Hempstead, Herts.: Harvester Wheatsheaf.

England, H. (1986) *Social Work as Art*, London: Allen and Unwin.

Ericson, R.V., Baranek, P.M. and Chan, J.B.L. (1987) *Visualizing Deviance*, Milton Keynes: Open University Press.

—— (1989) *Negotiating Control*, Milton Keynes: Open University Press.

—— (1991) *Representing Order*, Milton Keynes: Open University Press.

Etzioni, A. (ed.) (1969) *The Semi-Professions and their Organization*, New York: The Free Press.

Evans, H. (1978) *Pictures on a Page: Photo-journalism, Graphics and Picture-editing*, London: Heinemann.

—— (1983) *Good Times, Bad Times*, London: Weidenfeld and Nicholson.

Fowler, R. (1991) *Language in the News*, London: Routledge.

Fox (1990) *Report of the Panel of Inquiry into the Death of Stephanie Fox*, London: London Borough of Wandsworth.

Franklin, B. and Murphy, D. (1991) *What News? The Market, Politics and the Local Press*, London: Routledge.

Franklin, B. and Parton, N. (eds) (1991) *Social Work, the Media and Public Relations*, London: Routledge.

Frazer, E. (1987) 'Teenage girls reading *Jackie*', *Media, Culture and Society*, 9: 407–25.

Freidson, E. (1986) *Professional Powers*, Chicago: University of Chicago Press.

Fry, A. (1987) *Media Matters. Social Work, the Press and Broadcasting*, Wallington, Surrey: Community Care/Reed Business Publishing.

—— (1991) 'Reporting social work: a view from the newsroom', in B. Franklin and N. Parton (eds) *Social Work, the Media and Public Relations*, London: Routledge.

Galtung, J. and Ruge, M. (1965) 'The structure of foreign news: the presentation of the Congo, Cuba and Cyprus crises in four foreign newspapers', *International Journal of Peace Research*, 1: 64–90 (reprinted in S. Cohen and J. Young (eds) (1981) *The Manufacture of News: Deviance, Social Problems and the Mass Media* (revised second edition), London: Constable).

Glasgow University Media Group (1976) *Bad News*, London: Routledge and Kegan Paul.

—— (1980) *More Bad News*, London: Routledge and Kegan Paul.

—— (1985) *War and Peace News*, Milton Keynes: Open University Press.

Golding, P. (1991) 'Do-gooders on display: social work, public attitudes and the mass media', in B. Franklin and N. Parton (eds) *Social Work, the Media and Public Relations*, London: Routledge.

Golding, P. and Middleton, S. (1982) *Images of Welfare: Press and Public Attitudes to Poverty*, London: Martin Robertson.

Gordon, P. and Rosenberg, D. (1989) *Daily Racism: the Press and Black People in Britain*, London: The Runnymede Trust.

Graham, H. (1983) 'Caring: a labour of love', in J. Finch and D. Groves (eds) *A Labour of Love: Women, Work and Caring*, London: Routledge.

Griffiths, R. (1988) *Community Care: Agenda for Action*, London: HMSO.

Gunter, B. (1992) 'Learning from television', unpublished paper presented to the British Association Science Festival.

Hale, C. (1992) 'Crime and penal policy', in N. Manning and R. Page (eds) *Social Policy Review 4*, Canterbury, Kent: Social Policy Association.

Hall, S. (1981) 'The determination of news photographs', in S. Cohen and J. Young (eds) *The Manufacture of News: Deviance, Social Problems and the Mass Media* (revised second edition), London: Constable.

Hall, S., Crichter, C., Jefferson, T., Clarke, J. and Roberts, B. (1978) *Policing the Crisis: Mugging, the State and Law and Order*, London: Macmillan.

Hallett, C. (1989) 'Child abuse inquiries and public policy', in O. Stevenson (ed.) *Child Abuse: Public Policy and Professional Practice*, Hemel Hempstead, Herts.: Harvester Wheatsheaf.

Halliday, T. (1987) *Beyond Monopoly*, Chicago: University of Chicago Press.

Hartley, D. (1982) *Understanding News*, London: Methuen.

Hearn, J. (1982) 'Notes on patriarchy, professionalization and the semi-professions', *Sociology*, 16: 184–202.

Henry (1987) *Whose Child? The Report of the Public Inquiry into the Death of Tyra Henry*, London: London Borough of Lambeth.

Hollingsworth, M. (1985) *The Press and Political Dissent*, London: Pluto Press.

Holme, A. and Maizels, J. (1978) *Social Workers and Volunteers*, London: Allen and Unwin/British Association of Social Workers.

Howarth, V. (1991) 'Social work and the media: pitfalls and possibilities', in B. Franklin and N. Parton (eds) *Social Work, the Media and Public Relations*, London: Routlege.

Howe, D. (1992) 'Child abuse and the bureaucratization of social work', *Sociological Review*, 38: 491–508.

Hudson, B. (1992) 'Quasi-markets in health and social care in Britain: can the public sector respond?' *Policy and Politics*, 20, 131–42.

Hughes, E.C. (1971) 'Mistakes at work', in E.C. Hughes (ed.) *The Sociological Eye: Selected Papers on Work, Self and the Study of Society*, Chicago: Aldine/Atherton.

Hugman, R. (1991) *Power in Caring Professions*, London: Macmillan.

Illsley, P. (1989) *The Drama of Cleveland*, London: Campaign for Press and Broadcasting Freedom.

James, N. (1989) 'Emotional labour: skills and work in the social regulation of feeling', *Sociological Review*, 37, 1: 15–42.

Jameson, D. (1989) *Touched by Angels*, London: Penguin Books.

—— (1990) *The Last of the Hot Metal Men*, London: Penguin Books.

Jamous, H. and Peloille, B. (1970) 'Changes in the French university-hospital system', in J. Jackson (ed.) *Professions and Professionalization*, Cambridge: Cambridge University Press.

Johnson, N. (1990) *Reconstructing the Welfare State*, Hemel Hempstead, Herts.: Harvester Wheatsheaf.

Johnson, T. (1972) *Professions and Power*, London: Macmillan/British Sociological Association.

—— (1977) 'Professions and the class structure', in R. Scase (ed.) *Industrial Society: Class, Cleavage and Control*, London: Allen and Unwin.

Karpf, A. (1988) *Doctoring the Media*, London: Routledge.

Keith Lucas, A. (1972) *Giving and Taking Help*, Chapel Hill, NC: University of North Carolina Press.

Kingdon, J. (1984) *Agendas, Alternatives and Public Policies*, Boston: Little Brown and Co.

Knight, D. and Willmott, H. (eds) (1986) *Gender and the Labour Process*, Aldershot, Hants.: Gower.

Leighton, N. (1985) 'Personal and professional values – marriage or divorce?', in D. Watson (ed.) *A Code of Ethics for Social Work: the Second Step*, London: Routledge.

Levy, A. and Kahan, B. (1991) *The Pindown Experience and the Protection of Children*, Stafford: Staffordshire County Council.

McQuail, D. (1987) *Mass Communications Theory* (second edition), London: Sage.

McRobbie, A. (1982) '*Jackie*: an ideology of adolescent femininity', in B. Waites, T. Bennet and G.L. Martin (eds), *Popular Culture: Past and Present*, London: Croom Helm.

Manning, N. and Page, R. (eds) (1992) *Social Policy Review 4*, Canterbury, Kent: Social Policy Association.

Media Research Group (1987) *Media Coverage of London Councils*, London: Media Research Group, Goldsmith's College, University of London.

Morley, D. (1986) *Family Television: Cultural Power and Domestic Leisure*, London: Comedia.

Morrison, D. and Tumber, H. (1988) *Journalists at War*, London: Sage.

Napoli, J. and Napoli, L. (1990) 'The ethnic voice: heard, even seen . . . but only rarely read', *British Journalism Review*, 1, 2: 22–9.

National Institute for Social Work (NISW) (1982) *Social Workers: Their Role and Tasks* (the Barclay Report), London: Bedford Square Press.

National Society for the Prevention of Cruelty to Children (NSPCC) (1992) *A Short History*, London: NSPCC.

Nava, M. (1988) 'Cleveland and the press; outrage and anxiety in the reporting of child abuse', *Feminist Review*, 28: 103–21.

Negrine, R. (1989) *Politics and the Mass Media in Britain*, London: Routledge.

Northumbria Probation Service (1992) *The Dog That Finally Barked: the Tyneside Disturbances of 1991; a Probation Perspective*, Newcastle-upon-Tyne: Northumbria Probation Service.

Oxford Dictionary of the Christian Church (1974) (second edition) F.L. Cross and E.A. Livingstone (eds), Oxford: Oxford University Press.

Parkin, F. (1979) *Marxism and Class Theory: a Bourgeois Critique*, London: Tavistock.

Parry, N. and Parry, J. (1979) 'Social work, professionalism and the state', in N. Parry, M. Rustin and C. Satyamurti (eds) *Social Work, Welfare and the State*, London: Edward Arnold.

Parry, N., Rustin, M. and Satyamurti, C. (1979) *Social Work, Welfare and the State*, London: Edward Arnold.

Parton, C. and Parton, N. (1989) 'Child protection: the law and dangerousness', in O. Stevenson (ed.) *Child Abuse: Public Policy and Professional Practice*, Hemel Hempstead, Herts.: Harvester Wheatsheaf.

Parton, N. (1985) *The Politics of Child Abuse*, London: Macmillan.

—— (1991) *Governing the Family*, London: Macmillan.

Phillipson, C. (1992) 'Challenging the "spectre of old age": community care for older people in the 1990s', in N. Manning and R. Page (eds) *Social Policy Review 4*, Canterbury, Kent: Social Policy Association.

Philo, G. (1990) *Seeing and Believing: the Influence of Television*, London: Routledge.

Ruddock, M. (1991) 'A receptacle for public anger', in B. Franklin and N. Parton (eds) *Social Work, the Media and Public Relations*, London: Routledge.

Russell Hochschild, A. (1983) *The Managed Heart*, Berkeley, Calif.: University of California Press.

Sarfati Larson, M. (1977) *The Rise of Professionalism: a Sociological Analysis*, Berkeley, Calif.: University of California Press.

Satyamurti, C. (1981) *Occupational Survival*, Oxford: Basil Blackwell.

Schlesinger, P., Tumber, H. and Murdock, G. (1991) 'The media politics of crime and criminal justice', *British Journal of Sociology*, 42, 3: 397–420.

Schudson, M. (1989) 'The sociology of news production', *Media, Culture and Society*, 11, 3: 263–82.

Searle, C. (1987) 'Your daily dose: racism and the *Sun*', *Race and Class*, 29: 55–71.

Seymour-Ure, C. (1991) *The British Press and Broadcasting Since 1945*, London: Basil Blackwell.

Shaw, I. (1993) 'Centralization of power and decentralization of responsibility in the administration of public policy in Britain – the experience of health and the personal social services', unpublished paper delivered to the International Conference on the Public Sphere, University of Salford.

Simpson, R. and Simpson, I. (1969) 'Women and bureaucracy in the semi-professions', in A. Etzioni (ed.) *The Semi-Professions and their Organization*, New York: The Free Press.

Smith, P. (1992) *The Emotional Labour of Nursing*, London: Macmillan.

Smyth, G. (1990) 'Pressing our case: presenting probation work through the media', *Probation Journal*, 37, 4: 171–5.

Snow, R. (1994) 'Media and social order in everyday life', in M. Aldridge and N. Hewitt (eds) *Controlling Broadcasting: Policy and Practice in North America and Europe*, Manchester: Manchester University Press.

Soothill, K. and Walby, S. (1991) *Sex Crime in the News*, London: Routledge.

Stevenson, O. (ed.) (1989) *Child Abuse: Public Policy and Professional Practice*, Hemel Hempstead, Herts.: Harvester Wheatsheaf.

Thomas, W.I. (1932) *The Child in America*, New York: Alfred Knopf.

Toren, N. (1972) *Social Work: the Case of a Semi-Profession*, Beverly Hills, Calif.: Sage.

Tuchman, G. (1972) 'Objectivity as strategic ritual: an examination of newsman's notions of objectivity', *American Journal of Sociology*, 77, 4: 660–79.

—— (1978) *Making News: a Study in the Construction of Reality*, New York: The Free Press.

Tunstall, J. (1971) *Journalists at Work*, London: Constable.

van Dijk, T. (1991) *Racism and the Press*, London: Routledge.

Waddington, P. (1986) 'Mugging as a moral panic: a question of proportion', *British Journal of Sociology*, 37, 2: 245–59.

Waine, B. (1992) 'The voluntary sector: the Thatcher years', in N. Manning and R. Page (eds) *Social Policy Review 4*, Canterbury, Kent: Social Policy Association.

Walder, L. (1991) 'Public relations and social services: a view from the statutory sector', in B. Franklin and N. Parton (eds) *Social Work, the Media and Public Relations*, London: Routledge.

Walker, N. (1992) 'The *ex-parte* injunction as press gag: a cause for concern' *Journalists' Fellowship Programme Research Paper*, Oxford: Queen Elizabeth House.

Walters, R. (1991) 'The act of teaching', unpublished paper, University of Lancaster.

Watson, D. (ed.) (1985) *A Code of Ethics for Social Work: the Second Step*, London: Routledge.

Welsh, T. and Greenwood, W. (1992) *McNae's Essential Law for Journalists* (twelfth edition), London: Butterworth.

Wilding, P. (1992) 'The public sector in the 1980s', in N. Manning and R. Page (eds) *Social Policy Review 4*, Canterbury, Kent: Social Policy Association.

Witz, A. (1992) *Professions and Patriarchy*, London: Routledge.

Worcester, R. (1991) 'Who buys what and why?' *British Journalism Review*, 2, 4: 46–52.

Wroe, A. (1988) 'Social work, child abuse and the press' *Social Work Monographs 66*, Norwich: University of East Anglia.

Index

Abbott, P. 197
ACOP *see* Association of Chief
    Officers of Probation
ADSS *see* Association of Directors of
    Social Services
advertorial *see* placed news
Agence France Presse 26
Aldridge, M. 145
Allan, G. 199
Asian Times 154
Association of Chief Officers of
    Probation (ACOP) vii, ix, 121,
    123, 124, 130, 131, 135
Association of Directors of Social
    Services (ADSS) ix, 16, 163, 206,
    219

Bamford, T. 174
Barclay Committee 174–8, 186, 214
    see also NISW
Barclay, Peter 174 *see also* Barclay
    Committee, NISW
Barnardo's (children's charity) 82
BASW *see* British Association of
    Social Workers
Beck, Frank *see* Frank Beck case
Becker, H. 34, 71
Beckford, Jasmine *see* Jasmine
    Beckford case
Bevins, A. 31
Boateng, Janet 45, 46, 47, 49, 67
Bolger, S. 177
Bottomley, Virginia 78, 85, 87, 89
Boyd, A. 19–20, 24, 25, 33, 40
Bradford *Telegraph and Argus*, 15

Bradford social services department
    141, 221
Brawley, E. 201, 203
Brent social services department 158
Brewer, C. 186
Brighton *Evening Argus* 148, 165
British Association of Social
    Workers (BASW) ix, 44, 47, 48,
    73, 81, 85, 136, 163, 165, 169,
    174, 175, 176, 192, 194, 206,
    215–16, 220
British Journal of Social Work vii,
    195
broadcasting: 34, 157, 168, 170,
    171–2, 203; British Broadcasting
    Corporation 18, 132–3, 153,
    206–7; BBC news 21; British Sky
    Broadcasting (BSkyB) 12;
    Independent Television
    Commission 14; legal framework
    34, 171–2, 206–7, 217; television
    13, 14, 21, 27, 96, 107, 121, 137,
    145, 153, 156, 166, 217, 222;
    Independent Television News
    (ITN) 21, 121; radio 132–3, 137,
    153, 156, 222
Broadcasting Act 1990 172, 206,
    207, 217
Butler Sloss, Mrs Justice 96, 205,
    206 *see also* Kimberley Carlile
    case

Calcutt, Sir David 15 *see also* Cm
    1102 and Cm 2135
Calcutt Report 15; *see also* Cm 1102